Hilary McClafferty (Ed.)

Pediatric Integrative Medicine:
An Emerging Field of Pediatrics

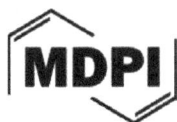

MDPI

This book is a reprint of the special issue that appeared in the online open access journal *Children* (ISSN 2227-9067) from 2014–2015 (available at: http://www.mdpi.com/journal/children/special_issues/pediatric_integrative_medicine).

Guest Editor
Hilary McClafferty
University of Arizona
Center for Integrative Medicine
3055 N. Campbell Ave. Suite 113
Tucson, AZ 85719
USA

Editorial Office
MDPI
Klybeckstrasse 64
Basel, Switzerland

Publisher
Shu-Kun Lin

Managing Editor
Delia Costache

1. Edition 2015

MDPI • Basel • Beijing • Wuhan

ISBN 978-3-03842-062-0 (Hbk)
ISBN 978-3-03842-063-7 (PDF)

.

Table of Contents

About the Editor

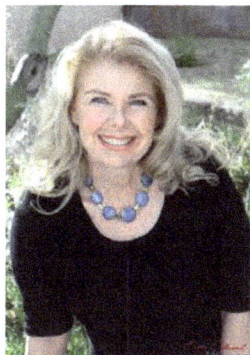

Hilary McClafferty, MD, FAAP is Director of the Pediatric Integrative Medicine in Residency program, and Interim Director of the Fellowship at the Arizona Center for Integrative Medicine, University of Arizona, Tucson. She received her medical degree from the University of Michigan, Ann Arbor, Michigan, and completed pediatric residency training at Northwestern Children's Memorial Hospital in Chicago, Illinois, and at the University of Arizona in Tucson, Arizona. She is fellowship trained in pediatric emergency medicine through The Children's Hospital, Denver, Colorado, certified in clinical hypnosis, and trained in medical acupuncture through the University of California, Los Angeles/ Helm's Medical Institute. She is founder of the Center for Women and Children's Integrative Medicine, a private consult practice in Chapel Hill, North Carolina. Dr. McClafferty Chairs the Executive Committee of the American Academy of Pediatrics Section on Integrative Medicine and the Special Interest Group for Physician Health and Wellness for the American Academy of Pediatrics. She led development of the first Clinical Report on Physician Health and Wellness for the Academy in 2014. Special interests include pediatric integrative medicine, mind-body medicine, interprofessional models in integrative healthcare, and physician health and wellness. She writes and speaks nationally on integrative medicine topics.

List of Contributors

Michelle G. Brenner: Eastern Virginia Medical School, Children's Hospital of the King's Daughters, Norfolk, VA 23507, USA

Audrey J. Brooks: Arizona Center for Integrative Medicine, University of Arizona College of Medicine, Tucson, AZ 85724, USA

Meredith Brooks: Department of Anesthesiology and Pain Medicine, Pediatric Anesthesiology, Stanford University, 300 Pasteur Dr. Stanford, CA 94304, USA

Melanie L. Brown: Department of Pediatrics, University of Chicago Comer Children's Hospital, Chicago, IL 60637, USA

Sally Dodds: Psychiatry and Medicine, University of Arizona College of Medicine, Tucson, AZ 85724, USA

Jeanne A. Drisko: Program in Integrative Medicine, University of Kansas Medical Center, Kansas City, KS, 66160, USA

Anna Esparham: Program in Integrative Medicine, University of Kansas Medical Center, Kansas City, KS, 66160, USA

Randall G. Evans: Program in Integrative Medicine, University of Kansas Medical Center, Kansas City, KS, 66160, USA

Hillary A. Franke: Department of Pediatrics, Section of Pediatric Critical Care, University of Arizona , Tucson, AZ 85716, USA

Paige Frazer: Community Faculty, Eastern Virginia Medical School, Children's Hospital of the King's Daughters, Norfolk, VA 23507, USA

Brenda Golianu: Department of Anesthesiology and Pain Medicine, Pediatric Anesthesiology, Stanford University, 300 Pasteur Dr. Stanford, CA 94304, USA

Pamela Kaiser: National Pediatric Hypnosis Training Institute (NPHTI), Private Practice, 1220 University Drive, Suite #104, Menlo Park, CA 94025, USA

Daniel P. Kohen: National Pediatric Hypnosis Training Institute (NPHTI), Developmental-Behavioral Pediatrics, Partners-in-Healing of Minneapolis, 10505 Wayzata Boulevard, Suite #200, Minnetonka, MN 55305, USA

Patricia Lebensohn: Arizona Center for Integrative Medicine, University of Arizona College of Medicine, Tucson, AZ 85724, USA

Victoria Maizes: Arizona Center for Integrative Medicine, University of Arizona College of Medicine, Tucson, AZ 85724, USA

John D. Mark: Pediatric Pulmonary Medicine, Lucile Packard Children's Hospital, Stanford University School of Medicine, Palo Alto, CA 94305, USA

Hilary McClafferty: Arizona Center for Integrative Medicine, University of Arizona College of Medicine, Tucson, AZ 85724, USA

Sanghamitra M. Misra: Academic General Pediatrics, Baylor College of Medicine, 6701 Fannin Street CCC 1540, Houston, TX 77030, USA

Ujjwal Ramtekkar: Mercy Children's Hospital, 621 S. New Ballas Road, Suite 693A, Saint Louis, MO 63141, USA

Amelia Villagomez: University of Arizona, 2800 E. Ajo Way Suite 300, Tucson, AZ 85713, USA

Leigh E. Wagner: Program in Integrative Medicine, University of Kansas Medical Center, Kansas City, KS, 66160, USA

Joy A. Weydert: Department of Pediatrics, University of Kansas Medical Center, 3901 Rainbow Blvd., MS 4004 Kansas City, KS 66160, USA

Graciela M. G. Wilcox: Department of Pediatrics, University of Arizona, Tucson, AZ 85724, USA

Ann Ming Yeh: Pediatric Gastroenterology, Stanford University, 750 Welch Road, Suite 116, Palo Alto CA 94304, USA

Integrative Pediatrics: Looking Forward

Hilary McClafferty

Abstract: Increase in the prevalence of disease and illness has dramatically altered the landscape of pediatrics. As a result, there is a demand for pediatricians with new skills and a sharper focus on preventative health. Patient demand and shifting pediatric illness patterns have accelerated research in the field of pediatric integrative medicine. This emerging field can be defined as healing-oriented medicine that considers the whole child, including all elements of lifestyle and family health. It is informed by evidence and carefully weighs all appropriate treatment options. This Special Issue of *Children*, containing a collection of articles written by expert clinicians, represents an important educational contribution to the field. The goal of the edition is to raise awareness about integrative topics with robust supporting evidence, and to identify areas where more research is needed.

Reprinted from *Children*. Cite as: McClafferty, H. Integrative Pediatrics: Looking Forward. *Children* **2015**, *2*, 63-65.

Increase in the prevalence of diseases such as attention deficit disorder, obesity, diabetes, metabolic syndrome, autism, cancer, chronic pain, mental illness, asthma, and other inflammatory mediated illnesses has dramatically altered the landscape of pediatrics, impacting progressively younger age groups [1]. Subsequently, today's children face serious health challenges, creating a demand for pediatricians with new skills and a sharper focus on preventive health. Limited treatment options, a desire to protect their child's health, and a perceived lack of support from conventional clinicians have caused many parents to turn to complementary medicine. Widely published statistics indicate that an estimated 12% of children use complementary therapies, with prevalence increasing to 50% in children living with chronic illness. Use often occurs without disclosure to the clinician for fear of negative repercussions [2]. Patient demand and shifting pediatric illness patterns have accelerated research in the field of pediatric integrative medicine. This emerging field can be defined as healing oriented medicine that considers the whole child, including all elements of lifestyle and family health. It is informed by evidence and carefully weighs all appropriate treatment options.

Interest in integrative pediatrics has grown relatively quickly, in step with recommendations from the Institute of Medicine for increased education and training in the field to meet consumer demands for information on evidence-based complementary medicine [3]. The American Academy of Pediatrics (AAP) was an early supporter of the field, endorsing a Provisional Section on Complementary and Integrative Medicine in 2005. Full AAP Section status was earned in 2009 [4]. The name was simplified to the Section on Integrative Medicine (SOIM) in 2011, mirroring national streamlining of nomenclature in the field. Surveys of AAP members have indicated high interest in integrative pediatrics [5], yet, to date, relatively few educational opportunities exist. For example, a national survey of academic pediatric institutions in 2012 by Vohra, *et al.* [6] identified integrative pediatric programs at only 16 of 143 academic pediatric programs in 2012.

This special edition of *Children*, containing a collection of articles written by expert clinicians, represents an important educational contribution to the field. The goal of the edition is to raise awareness about integrative topics with robust supporting evidence, and to identify areas where more research is needed. Toxic stress, attention deficit disorder, vitamin D in children's health, clinical hypnosis in children and adolescents, acupuncture for pediatric pain, integrative approaches to reflux, functional dyspepsia, and inflammatory bowel disease are some of the topics represented. Multiple case studies are included to demonstrate clinical application of integrative treatments.

Another development in the educational arena is the *Pediatric Integrative Medicine in Residency* (PIMR) program, a 100-hour online curriculum developed at the University of Arizona Center for Integrative Medicine. Designed to be embedded into conventional residency training, the program is halfway through a three-year national pilot phase at five US pediatric residencies: University of Arizona Department of Pediatrics, Stanford Children's Health, University of Chicago Comer Children's Hospital, Eastern Virginia Medical School/Children's Hospital of the King's Daughters, and the University of Kansas Department of Pediatrics, involving more than 300 pediatric residents and a dozen faculty. Early adopters of the program include Vanderbilt University School of Medicine Department of Pediatrics, Cardinal Glennon Children's Medical Center, and the University of New Mexico Department of Pediatrics. The PIMR educational curriculum covers foundations of integrative medicine, including nutrition, mind-body medicine, physical activity, sleep, environment and health, and an introduction to whole medical systems. It also uses case-based teaching to introduce integrative approaches to common clinical conditions.

Although progress in the field of integrative pediatrics is evident, real obstacles exist, among them being unequal insurance reimbursement for children's health issues [7,8], lack of research funding, skepticism from colleagues and administrators, compressed time during office visits, and competition from pharmaceutical companies. Recognition of these obstacles is important, yet so is acknowledgment of the relative lack of progress in prevention and treatment of complex pediatric conditions, such as obesity and autism, highlighting a call for new approaches. In reality, given the prevalence of integrative medicine use in children, even skeptics will require understanding of the potential risks and benefits of integrative treatments, in order to be prepared to direct patients and their families toward reliable resources.

It is possible that the most important benefit of integrative pediatrics is its potential for reduction in health care costs. Imagine the financial implications of a generation of children where the norm is healthy weight, mastery of self-regulation skills, avoidance of harmful environmental toxins, and the ability to apply evidence-based approaches to combat preventable chronic illness. Integrative pediatrics embraces each of these areas as fundamental to good health. In the search for models of medical care tailored to the children of today, I believe integrative medicine holds significant promise.

Hilary McClafferty, MD, FAAP

Conflicts of Interest

The authors declare no conflict of interest.

References

1. Kemper, K.J.; Vohra, S.; Walls, R.; Task Force on Complementary and Alternative Medicine; Provisional Section on Complementary, Holistic, and Integrative Medicine. American Academy of Pediatrics. The use of complementary and alternative medicine in pediatrics. *Pediatrics* **2008**, *122*, 1374–1386, doi:10.1542/peds.2008-2173. PMID: 19047261
2. Birdee, G.S.; Phillips, R.S.; Davis, R.B.; Gardiner, P. Factors associated with pediatric use of complementary and alternative medicine. *Pediatrics* **2010**, *125*, 249–256, doi:10.1542/peds.2009-1406. Epub 2010 Jan 25. PMID: 20100769
3. Institute of Medicine. *Report, Complementary and Alternative Medicine in the United States*; National Academies Press: Washington, DC, USA, 2005. Available online: http://www.iom.edu/reports/2005/complementary-and-alternative-medicine-in-the-united-states.aspx (accessed on 28 December 2014).
4. American Academy of Pediatrics Section on Integrative Medicine. Available online: http://www2.aap.org/sections/chim/ (accessed on 5 January 2015).
5. Kemper, K.J.; O'Connor, K.G. Pediatricians' recommendations for complementary and alternative medical (CAM) therapies. *Ambul. Pediatr.* **2004**, *4*, 482–487. PMID: 15548098
6. Vohra, S.; Surette, S.; Rosen, L.D.; Gardiner, P.; Kemper, K.J. Pediatric integrative medicine: Pediatrics' newest subspecialty? *BMC Pediatr.* **2012**, *15*, 123, doi:10.1186/1471-2431-12-123. PMID: 22894682
7. Cheng, T.L.; Wise, P.H.; Halfon, N. Quality health care for children and the affordable health care act: A voltage drop checklist. *Pediatrics* **2014**, *134*, 794–802. PMID: 25225140
8. Howell, E.M.; Kenney, G.M. The impact of the Medicaid/CHIP expansions on children: A synthesis of the evidence. *Med. Care Res. Rev.* **2012**, *69*, 372–396, doi:10.1177/1077558712437245. Epub 2012 Mar 26. PMID: 22451618

4

Toxic Stress: Effects, Prevention and Treatment

Hillary A. Franke

Abstract: Children who experience early life toxic stress are at risk of long-term adverse health effects that may not manifest until adulthood. This article briefly summarizes the findings in recent studies on toxic stress and childhood adversity following the publication of the American Academy of Pediatrics (AAP) Policy Report on the effects of toxic stress. A review of toxic stress and its effects is described, including factors of vulnerability, resilience, and the relaxation response. An integrative approach to the prevention and treatment of toxic stress necessitates individual, community and national focus.

Reprinted from *Children*. Cite as: Franke, H.A. Toxic Stress: Effects, Prevention and Treatment. *Children* **2014**, *1*, 390-402.

1. Introduction

Stress is a term commonly used to describe the response to the demands encountered on a daily basis throughout one's lifetime, and it is related to both positive experiences and negative experiences. Stressors are agents that produce stress. Stressors may be physical, emotional, environmental or theoretical, and all may equally affect the body's stress response. The stress response, also known as the "fight or flight" response or general adaptation syndrome, comprises the physiologic changes that occur with any encounter of stress or perceived stress to the individual [1,2]. This stress response is a result of stimulation of the sympathetic nervous system resulting in a cascade of neuro-endocrine-immune responses, with reproducible physiologic effects that include an increase in respirations, heart rate, blood pressure, and overall oxygen consumption [3,4]. In most situations, the physiologic changes associated with the stress response are transient, with the body returning to its baseline state when the stressor is removed. Toxic stress responses include a prolonged or permanent abnormal physiologic response to a stressor with risk of end organ dysfunction [5,6]. Toxic stress can affect anyone, and children are no exception.

Childhood toxic stress is severe, prolonged, or repetitive adversity with a lack of the necessary nurturance or support of a caregiver to prevent an abnormal stress response [5]. This abnormal stress response consists of a derangement of the neuro-endocrine-immune response resulting in prolonged cortisol activation and a persistent inflammatory state, with failure of the body to normalize these changes after the stressor is removed [6,7]. Children who experience early life toxic stress are at risk of long-term adverse health effects that may not manifest until adulthood. These adverse health effects include maladaptive coping skills, poor stress management, unhealthy lifestyles, mental illness and physical disease [5,6,8–13].

In January 2012, the AAP published a policy statement on the effects of toxic stress and childhood adversity using an ecobiodevelopmental framework to approach this important public health concern [8]. This framework acknowledges the interactions of personal experiences, environmental influences, and genetic predispositions that shape the learning and behavior of an individual across his or her lifespan. The AAP put out a call to action, including the following recommendations: a need for understanding that lifelong disparities are determined by social, behavioral and economic determinants; proper training of all healthcare providers in the effects of toxic stress; and ongoing advocacy by pediatric providers. The medical home becomes an important venue for thorough anticipatory guidance, active screening for at-risk children, knowledge of local resources, identification and implementation of interventions to decrease sources of toxic stress, and development of comprehensive treatment plans for mitigation of toxic stress effects [8,9].

2. Stress—Positive, Tolerable, Toxic

Early childhood experiences play a large role in how the brain develops and functions. Interactions with the child and his or her environment affect long-term learning, behavior, and health. Healthy brain architecture relies on responsive caregivers and positive relationships that help children learn to handle stressful experiences. In general, the stress response is a physiologic response to an adverse event or demanding circumstance and includes biochemical changes to the neurologic, endocrine, and immune systems.

2.1. Positive Stress

A positive stress response is a normal stress response and is essential for the growth and development of a child. Positive stress responses are infrequent, short-lived, and mild. The child is supported through this stressful event with strong social and emotional buffers such as reassurance and parental protection. The child gains motivation and resilience from every positive stress response, and the biochemical reactions that occur with such a stressful event return to baseline [5]. Examples include meeting new people or learning a new task.

2.2. Tolerable Stress

Tolerable stress responses are more severe, frequent or sustained. The body responds to a greater degree, and these biochemical responses have the potential to negatively affect brain architecture. Examples include divorce or the death of a loved one. In tolerable stress responses, once the adversity is removed, the brain and organs recover fully given the condition that the child is protected with responsive relationships and strong social and emotional support.

2.3. Toxic Stress

Toxic stress results in prolonged activation of the stress response, with a failure of the body to recover fully. It differs from a normal stress response in that there is a lack of caregiver support, reassurance, or emotional attachments. The insufficient caretaker support prevents the buffering of the stress response or the return of the body to baseline function. Examples of toxic stress include abuse, neglect, extreme poverty, violence, household dysfunction, and food scarcity. Caretakers with substance abuse or mental health conditions also predispose a child to a toxic stress response.

Exposure to less severe yet chronic, ongoing daily stressors can also be toxic to children [14]. Early life toxic stressors increase one's vulnerability to maladaptive health outcomes such as an unhealthy lifestyle, socioeconomic inequity, and poor health; however, these stressors do not solely predict or determine an adult's behavior or health [10,14].

3. Toxic Stress Effects

A child experiencing adversity is at risk of permanent changes to brain architecture, epigenetic alteration, and modified gene function. Implications for long-term health and developmental effects are critical, including increased risk for stress-related diseases [5,15]. The toxic stress response affects the neuroendocrine-immune network, and the response leads to a prolonged and abnormal cortisol response [6,7]. The resultant immune dysregulation, including a persistent inflammatory state, increases the risk and frequency of infections in children [16–18]. The toxic stress response is believed to play a role in the pathophysiology of depressive disorders, behavioral dysregulation, PTSD, and psychosis [13,19–25]. Adults who endured early childhood adversity also experience more physical illness and poor health outcomes [11,16–18,26,27]. These poor health outcomes are varied and include alcoholism, chronic obstructive pulmonary disease, depression, cancer, obesity, increase in suicide attempts, ischemic heart disease and myriad other disease processes [11,28,29]. A proposed model relating the effects of toxic stress to a potential increased risk of cancer suggest both a direct effect of stress on biological systems and an indirect effect of poor health behaviors as responses to stress [30].

Large longitudinal studies like the Adverse Childhood Experiences (ACE) study and the Coronary Artery Risk Development in Young Adults study show correlation with the number of ACE and the increased risk of multisystem health problems in a graded fashion [11,31]. Notably, low levels of parental warmth and affection with high levels of abuse had the highest multisystem health risk as adults. Inversely, strong parental warmth and affection during childhood was associated with less health risk in adulthood [31]. Maternal warmth appears to buffer toxic stressors, such as growing up in extreme poverty [31,32]. Maternal support may have a protective effect on childhood abuse, and it also appears to be a variable determining a positive response to therapies [33,34]. Ongoing familial support including maternal care and paternal protection have been shown to affect treatment response in situations of abuse and are more predictive of success than the type of the abuse experienced [33].

4. Resilience and Vulnerability

Resilience is the ability to properly adapt to adversity despite the conditions. It is dynamic and plays a large role in a toxic stress response. Not all individuals who experience repeated childhood adversity experience poor health, and resilience may provide a buffer. Resilience factors are numerous and change over time in an individual. Children with resilience have been identified as having the following characteristics: higher IQ, easy temperament, a perception of competence, a positive self concept, a realistic sense of control of the situation, empathy, and social problem solving skills [34–37]. Factors that predict resilience in children experiencing adversity include a solid relationship between the child and parent as well as a high quality relationship between the child and teacher [37]. Additional resilience factors identified include adequate social support, marriage quality, the physical and mental health of the parent, and the parent's sense of efficacy [33,34,37–39]. Prior adaptive behaviors that result in overcoming adversity strengthen resilience. Focus on early interventions to strengthen resilience factors may help to minimize a toxic stress response [28].

Factors believed to increase vulnerability to early toxic stress include an individual's increased sensitivity to both psychological and physiologic stress with a decreased resources for social and psychological support to help with stress coping skills [18]. Other sources of vulnerability may include poor social support, developmental delays, abusive parenting, and maladaptive behaviors in response to adversity [36].

5. Relaxation Response

Documented in the 1970s by Herbert Benson, the relaxation response is a state of decreased sympathetic nervous system activity that opposes the stress response [4,40]. Physiologic effects of the relaxation response include a reduction in respirations, heart rate, blood pressure, and oxygen consumption, with an increase in heart rate variability; these effects have been elicited regularly and repetitively with techniques including transcendental meditation, autogenic hypnosis, Zen and yoga, contention, sentic cycles, and progressive muscle relaxation [40]. Conscious effort and practice are indicated for achieving ongoing effects of the relaxation response, however many techniques require minimal instruction or practice to immediately produce the calming effects.

Techniques may be as simple and informal as repeating a word or phrase while sitting comfortably in a quiet area or taking several deep breaths [40,41]. Formal programs such as The Relaxation Response Resiliency Program (3RP) use adaptive coping mechanisms for chronic stress [42]. The 3RP uses components of a relaxation response strategy, stress coping, growth enhancement and inter-connectedness to address and promote resiliency, and this regimented approach may demonstrate benefit for individuals in communities with chronic stress [42]. Other techniques, such as biofeedback, guided imagery, and mindful awareness may take time to establish into routine. While techniques vary, there are four basic components that, when combined, produce the relaxation response; these include a repetitive sound or phrase, a passive attitude of disregard to distraction, relaxed positioning, and a quiet environment [40]. There are many ways to reach a state of relaxation response, and for best achievability and sustainability, the individual's preference to technique and resources such as time and financial investment for the technique must be taken into account.

The relaxation response has been effective as a tool for situations in which excessive sympathetic activity prevails, such as would be considered in exposures to toxic stress [40]. Children, their parents, family members and community members may benefit from awareness of the relaxation response, and these skills may help build resiliency for future stressors.

6. Unique Role of the Pediatrician to Address Toxic Stress

A pediatrician-led medical home has been identified by the AAP as an important venue to best identify risk factors, to prevent and reduce toxic stress, as well as to build resiliency in individuals and families [8]. Ideally, the pediatrician's perspective of childhood health that places focus on prevention, use of developmental milestones, and advocacy for a safe childhood experience makes for a broad base upon which to address toxic stress. Realistically, pediatricians have ever-increasing demands with decreasing time and resources, making this additional screening and treatment difficult, if not an impossible challenge. How does a pediatrician address these important needs for their patients and families? The pediatrician-led medical home requires resources in order to adequately provide standard of care and to also be able to meet the needs of individuals, family, and community with regards to toxic stress. This challenge to provide the care required for our nation, communities, and individuals does not have a simple answer. Programs in place that are successful will build awareness of need for programs throughout the country.

Some useful interventions as well as hardwired processes in the pediatrician's office may address toxic stress while not causing an enormous strain on already limited resources. For example, prioritizing the hardwiring of a toxic stress screening process upon entry of a patient to the exam room may be helpful. Posting handouts on instructions for breathing techniques, a list of free smart phone applications on biofeedback, or websites for stress reduction may give patients and families an awareness of relaxation. Some topics may be discussed during certain well child visits if time permits. A monitor in the waiting area with topics of childhood health may include toxic stress as a topic. Pediatricians may start with simple steps and as each technique is hardwired one may consider tackling another.

7. Screening for Toxic Stress

A child risks maladaptive stress responses when exposed to childhood adversity and toxic stress. The first several years of life are sensitive periods of time for increased neuroplasticity, after which it begins to wane [43,44]. If primary preventive measures are implemented during the early, sensitive windows of development, appropriate stress responses to adversity may result. Screening is a means to identify those children who would benefit from both preventive measures and, if need be, therapeutic interventions.

Factors that place a child at risk of maltreatment overlap those with risk of toxic stress, and the AAP recommends screening for factors such as social isolation, poverty, unemployment, low educational achievement, single-parent home, non-biologically related male living in the home, and family or intimate partner violence, young parental age, and parent factors such as low self-esteem, substance abuse, and depression [45]. Protective factors for child maltreatment may also be useful to attenuate a toxic stress risk, and some of these factors include presence of a caring and supportive adult, positive family changes, structured school environment, access to healthcare and social services, involvement with religious community or extracurricular organized activity [45]. The AAP has not as of yet identified a specific screening tool to be used for toxic stress or one to be incorporated within usual screening protocols such as the developmental milestones.

Social-emotional screening has been shown to predict behavioral problems and would fit with the need to identify children at risk of toxic stress [46]. Promise has been seen with use of the Ages and Stages Questionnaires: Social-Emotional screening tool, however broad use within multiple pediatric settings is necessary [47].

8. Prevention of Toxic Stress

Toxic stress is a function of the absence of buffers to return the stress response to baseline, and it is important to consider preventive measures that promote positive environmental influences and interactions with supportive caretakers. Routine anticipatory guidance, which encourages positive parenting, strengthens support for families, and builds resilience, helps develop the buffers required to handle stress and avoid toxic stress. AAP resources such as *Bright Futures*, *Connected Kids*, *Medical Home* and "The Pediatrician's Role in Child Maltreatment Prevention" offer recommendations [45,48]. Preventive interventions should be focused on only those children at risk of adverse childhood events. Children screened and found to have no risk of toxic stress may actually experience a detrimental stress response to an intervention [37]. Preventive measures to improve resilience in the child are notable, as is focus on aiding assisting the caretaker. Targeting the caretaker's stressors and improving the caretaker's capacity to provide safe, stable and nurturing relationships may mitigate any toxic stress response in children [31,32].

9. Treatment of Toxic Stress

An integrative approach to manage and prevent stress in general may play a vital role in preventing and treating childhood toxic stress. Treatment of toxic stress requires timely intervention, and goals are to decrease stressors and the individual's response to stressors, to minimize vulnerability, and to strengthen resiliency. Treatment should be aimed at the needs of each individual. Toxic stress effects are widespread and involve community and implicate healthcare on a national level. Approach to the individual, the caretakers and immediate family, the community, and awareness at the national level are indicated.

9.1. Individual and Family

Helping children learn to shut off their stress response in a healthy manner is important, and multiple approaches can be used for this goal. Conventional approaches such as referral to social work, psychology, or psychiatry may be beneficial, however these interventions can be costly. If therapy is indicated, the type of therapy depends on the adversity experienced. Evidence supports the use of parent-child interaction therapy, child-parent psychotherapy, cognitive behavioral therapy, and trauma-focused psychotherapy for children showing signs of toxic stress [33,35].

Integrative approaches to the child include attenuating the stress response and building resiliency. Tapping into the relaxation response with breathing techniques, guided imagery, and biofeedback may be well received depending on the age of child and if different techniques are offered as options. Mindfulness-based stress reduction or mindfulness-based cognitive therapy are time-intensive therapies requiring an instructor with years of experience, but if available and feasible, may be beneficial as studies suggest decreased anxiety, improved mood, relief of psychological distress and strengthened wellbeing [49]. Biofeedback is an effective tool to decrease heart rate and respiratory rate, increase heart rate variability and improve pulmonary peak flows [50,51]. Patients are able to measure changes objectively, which may benefit those with a suspicion for integrative approaches. Patients with comorbidities such as asthma may profit from this relaxation modality by learning about their body's response to different input while also gaining the control to potentially halt exacerbations of illness. Other mind-body interventions shown to decrease stress include hypnosis, guided imagery, music therapy, and progressive muscle relaxation [52–58].

A systematic review of cortisol regulation in children demonstrated numerous interventions to decrease stress response. Interventions centered on the child or adolescent showing benefit included guided imagery, social and educational enrichment, and in-home sessions to develop language skills [59]. Interestingly, improved cortisol response was also seen in children when interventions focused solely on the child's caretaker [59]. Parenting classes, home visits to improve parenting practice, telephone support, family-based programs, access to social resources for parents, problem solving and information seeking skills, and peer support were beneficial [59]. A focus on the caretaker may be one part of the approach to reduce toxic stress risk. Having stable relationships so a child senses a safe environment is important to avoid toxic stress effects [60].

Teaching families these techniques for relaxation takes time and in a busy practice it may be difficult to accomplish. Using handouts and giving parents online resources may help spread information about the importance of stress reduction and give step-by-step instructions. Judicious use of the internet may supplement the pediatrician's current resources with further information including techniques to help build resiliency, to teach parents to establish healthy connections, and to identify tools to cope with chronic stressors. For example, helpguide.org addresses many topics including stress reduction, parenting and attachment, relationships, and child issues [61]. The American Institute of Stress has information and techniques for dealing with stressors in daily life, the workplace, and in certain family situations such as those in the military [62]. Biofeedback products are available online, with information for research studies available as well [63,64]. Mind-body topics are also available on medical websites and websites of integrative medicine organizations. Relaxation response techniques are being studied in the virtual environment, and individuals report that having an ability to personalize the virtual online environment as well as participate anonymously without judgment has been well received, and it is anticipated that future online experiences with mind-body medicine education will expand [65]. Numerous stress reduction applications for smart phones have been developed and many are free for download. Internet accessibility may not be available for all families in a pediatric practice, however summary handouts or referral to a public library may be feasible.

9.2. Community

Community-based interventions that strengthen neighborhood-level resources may be most effective in buffering the toxic stress response in children [60]. It is important to know what community resources, outreach programs, and active volunteer groups are in the area for your patients in which to become involved or if they could benefit from additional services. Groups may be willing to volunteer time and resources to use to improve the lives of children, only they may not be aware of this important issue. Looking to these groups and initiating contact about important pediatric topics may lead to change, and at the least will increase community awareness of toxic stress.

Positive environmental changes can improve childhood outcomes, even in extreme cases of adversity. Community based interventions have been shown to be effective and long-term follow up of children involved in interventional programs exhibit enduring behavior and health effects [28,66,67]. Early-intervention programs such as Head Start may affect a child's development and exposure to positive experiences while decreasing the adversity of hunger that many children would otherwise experience [6,44].

Community organized home visits may be a mechanism to lend support to caretakers in the natural home environment [28]. Caretaker skill building, including improving the caretaker's employability and resultant economic stability, is imperative for protecting children from toxic stress [60].

9.3. National

Early toxic stress affects our entire nation. The effects of early toxic stress are realized through adulthood, with large costs to the individual as well as to society. The potential exists to prevent adult-onset diseases by targeting and promoting healthy stress responses in childhood. National awareness of the effects of adverse childhood events allows further opportunity for interventions. Pediatricians are asked to involve schools, community, and government to help aid with toxic stress interventions [28]. Advocacy on a national level is imperative to lobby for funding of meaningful programs and to gain support, financially and otherwise for pediatric healthcare workers to appropriately and adequately screen for toxic stress in the office setting. The AAP is present at the national level and will continue to advocate for the better care of children, including awareness, prevention, and early treatment of toxic stress.

10. Conclusions

Toxic stress burdens society, and everyone is susceptible to its effects. Awareness of early childhood adversity risk and resultant downstream effects of toxic stress is key. Prevention must begin early with the targeting of at-risk populations. Protection of children from toxic stress requires a multi-faceted approach, including interventions that will target the child, the caretaker, and the environment. Strengthening the stability of the family as well as the community affords environmental protection against childhood effects of toxic stress. Use of proven stress reduction strategies is important, and many mind-body approaches are effective in eliciting the relaxation response. Appropriate management of the adolescent or adult patient with resultant health effects from toxic stress necessitates full knowledge of the long-term effects of the toxic stress response, including the need for stress reduction, coping techniques, and use of an integrative approach to therapy.

12

Conflicts of Interest

The author declares no conflict of interest.

References

1. Cannon, W.B. Bodily changes in pain, hunger, fear and rage, an account of recent researches into the function of emotional excitement; Hardpress Ltd: New York, NY, USA, 2013.
2. Selye, H. Forty years of stress research: principal remaining problems and misconceptions. *Can. Med. Assoc. J.* **1976**, *115*, 53–56.
3. Chrousos, G.P. The Concepts of Stress and Stress System Disorders: Overview of Physical and Behavioral Homeostasis. *JAMA* **1992**, *267*, 1244.
4. Dusek, J. A.; Benson, H. Mind-body medicine: a model of the comparative clinical impact of the acute stress and relaxation responses. *Minn. Med.* **2009**, *92*, 47–50.
5. National Scientific Council on the Developing Child. Excessive Stress Disrupts the Architecture of the Developing Brain: Working Paper 3. Updated Edition. www.developingchild.harvard.edu (accessed 1 May, 2014).
6. Johnson, S.B.; Riley, A.W.; Granger, D.A.; Riis, J. The Science of Early Life Toxic Stress for Pediatric Practice and Advocacy. *PEDIATRICS* **2013**, *131*, 319–327.
7. Wolf, J.M.; Miller, G.E.; Chen, E. Parent psychological states predict changes in inflammatory markers in children with asthma and healthy children. *Brain. Behav. Immun.* **2008**, *22*, 433–441.
8. Committee on Psychosocial Aspects of Child and Family Health, Committee on Early Childhood, Adoption, and Dependent Care, and Section on Developmental and Behavioral Pediatrics; Garner, A. S.; Shonkoff, J.P.; Siegel, B.S.; Dobbins, M.I.; Earls, M.F.; Garner, A.S.; McGuinn, L.; Pascoe, J.; Wood, D.L. Early Childhood Adversity, Toxic Stress, and the Role of the Pediatrician: Translating Developmental Science Into Lifelong Health. *PEDIATRICS* **2012**, *129*, e224–e231.
9. Shonkoff, J.P.; Garner, A.S.; THE COMMITTEE ON PSYCHOSOCIAL ASPECTS OF CHILD AND FAMILY HEALTH, COMMITTEE ON EARLY CHILDHOOD, ADOPTION, AND DEPENDENT CARE, AND SECTION ON DEVELOPMENTAL AND BEHAVIORAL PEDIATRICS; Siegel, B.S.; Dobbins, M.I.; Earls, M. F.; Garner, A.S.; McGuinn, L.; Pascoe, J.; Wood, D. L. The Lifelong Effects of Early Childhood Adversity and Toxic Stress. *PEDIATRICS* **2012**, *129*, e232–e246.
10. Shonkoff, J.P.; Boyce, W.T.; McEwen, B.S. Neuroscience, Molecular Biology, and the Childhood Roots of Health Disparities: Building a New Framework for Health Promotion and Disease Prevention. *JAMA* **2009**, *301*, 2252.
11. Felitti, V.J.; Anda, R.F.; Nordenberg, D.; Williamson, D.F.; Spitz, A.M.; Edwards, V.; Koss, M.P.; Marks, J.S. Relationship of Childhood Abuse and Household Dysfunction to Many of the Leading Causes of Death in Adults. *Am. J. Prev. Med. 14*, 245–258.
12. Yates, T.M. The Developmental Consequences of Child Emotional Abuse: A Neurodevelopmental Perspective. *J. Emot. Abuse* **2007**, *7*, 9–34.

13. Varese, F.; Smeets, F.; Drukker, M.; Lieverse, R.; Lataster, T.; Viechtbauer, W.; Read, J.; van Os, J.; Bentall, R. P. Childhood Adversities Increase the Risk of Psychosis: A Meta-analysis of Patient-Control, Prospective- and Cross-sectional Cohort Studies. *Schizophr. Bull.* **2012**, *38*, 661–671.

14. Odgers, C.L.; Jaffee, S.R. Routine Versus Catastrophic Influences on the Developing Child. *Annu. Rev. Public Health* **2013**, *34*, 29–48.

15. Bick, J.; Naumova, O.; Hunter, S.; Barbot, B.; Lee, M.; Luthar, S. S.; Raefski, A.; Grigorenko, E.L. Childhood adversity and DNA methylation of genes involved in the hypothalamus–pituitary–adrenal axis and immune system: Whole-genome and candidate-gene associations. *Dev. Psychopathol.* **2012**, *24*, 1417–1425.

16. Wyman, P.A.; Moynihan, J.; Eberly, S.; Cox, C.; Cross, W.; Jin, X.; Caserta, M.T. Association of family stress with natural killer cell activity and the frequency of illnesses in children. *Arch. Pediatr. Adolesc. Med.* **2007**, *161*, 228–234.

17. Caserta, M.T.; O'Connor, T.G.; Wyman, P.A.; Wang, H.; Moynihan, J.; Cross, W.; Tu, X.; Jin, X. The associations between psychosocial stress and the frequency of illness, and innate and adaptive immune function in children. *Brain. Behav. Immun.* **2008**, *22*, 933–940.

18. Fagundes, C.P.; Glaser, R.; Kiecolt-Glaser, J.K. Stressful early life experiences and immune dysregulation across the lifespan. *Brain. Behav. Immun.* **2013**, *27*, 8–12.

19. Carrion, V.G.; Weems, C.F.; Reiss, A.L. Stress Predicts Brain Changes in Children: A Pilot Longitudinal Study on Youth Stress, Posttraumatic Stress Disorder, and the Hippocampus. *PEDIATRICS* **2007**, *119*, 509–516.

20. Aguilera, M.; Arias, B.; Wichers, M.; Barrantes-Vidal, N.; Moya, J.; Villa, H.; van Os, J.; Ibáñez, M.I.; Ruipérez, M.A.; Ortet, G.; Fañanás, L. Early adversity and 5-HTT/BDNF genes: new evidence of gene–environment interactions on depressive symptoms in a general population. *Psychol. Med.* **2009**, *39*, 1425.

21. Heim, C.; Newport, D. J.; Mletzko, T.; Miller, A. H.; Nemeroff, C. B. The link between childhood trauma and depression: insights from HPA axis studies in humans. *Psychoneuroendocrinology* **2008**, *33*, 693–710.

22. Saveanu, R.V.; Nemeroff, C.B. Etiology of Depression: Genetic and Environmental Factors. *Psychiatr. Clin. North Am.* **2012**, *35*, 51–71.

23. McCrory, E.; de Brito, S.A.; Viding, E. The link between child abuse and psychopathology: A review of neurobiological and genetic research. *JRSM* **2012**, *105*, 151–156.

24. Matheson, S.L.; Shepherd, A.M.; Pinchbeck, R.M.; Laurens, K.R.; Carr, V.J. Childhood adversity in schizophrenia: a systematic meta-analysis. *Psychol. Med.* **2013**, *43*, 225–238.

25. Reavis, J. Adverse Childhood Experiences and Adult Criminality: How Long Must We Live before We Possess Our Own Lives? *Perm. J.* **2013**, *17*, 44–48.

26. Anda, R.F.; Felitti, V.J.; Bremner, J.D.; Walker, J.D.; Whitfield, C.; Perry, B.D.; Dube, S.R.; Giles, W.H. The enduring effects of abuse and related adverse experiences in childhood. A convergence of evidence from neurobiology and epidemiology. *Eur. Arch. Psychiatry Clin. Neurosci.* **2006**, *256*, 174–186.

27. Danese, A.; Moffitt, T.E.; Harrington, H.; Milne, B. J.; Polanczyk, G.; Pariante, C.M.; Poulton, R.; Caspi, A. Adverse Childhood Experiences and Adult Risk Factors for Age-Related Disease: Depression, Inflammation, and Clustering of Metabolic Risk Markers. *Arch. Pediatr. Adolesc. Med.* **2009**, *163*.

28. Garner, A. S. Home Visiting and the Biology of Toxic Stress: Opportunities to Address Early Childhood Adversity. *PEDIATRICS* **2013**, *132*, S65–S73.

29. Benjet, C.; Borges, G.; Medina-Mora, M. E.; Méndez, E. Chronic childhood adversity and stages of substance use involvement in adolescents. *Drug Alcohol Depend.* **2013**, *131*, 85–91.

30. Kelly-Irving, M.; Mabile, L.; Grosclaude, P.; Lang, T.; Delpierre, C. The embodiment of adverse childhood experiences and cancer development: potential biological mechanisms and pathways across the life course. *Int. J. Public Health* **2013**, *58*, 3–11.

31. Carroll, J.E.; Gruenewald, T.L.; Taylor, S.E.; Janicki-Deverts, D.; Matthews, K.; Seeman, T.E. Childhood abuse, parental warmth, and adult multisystem biological risk in the Coronary Artery Risk Development in Young Adults study. *Proc. Natl. Acad. Sci.* **2013**, *110*, 17149–17153.

32. Chen, E.; Miller, G.E.; Kobor, M.S.; Cole, S.W. Maternal warmth buffers the effects of low early-life socioeconomic status on pro-inflammatory signaling in adulthood. *Mol. Psychiatry* **2011**, *16*, 729–737.

33. Johnstone, J.M.; Carter, J.D.; Luty, S.E.; Mulder, R.T.; Frampton, C.M.; Joyce, P.R. Maternal care and paternal protection influence response to psychotherapy treatment for adult depression. *J. Affect. Disord.* **2013**, *149*, 221–229.

34. Cowen, E.L.; Wyman, P.A.; Work, W. C. Resilience in highly stressed urban children: concepts and findings. *Bull. N. Y. Acad. Med.* **1996**, *73*, 267–284.

35. Committee on Treatment of Posttraumatic Stress Disorder; Berg, A.O.; Breslau, N.; Goodman, S.N.; Lezak, M.D.; Matchar, D.B.; Mellman, T.A.; Spiegel, D.; Vega, W.A. *Treatment of PTSD: An Assessment of The Evidence*; Institution of Medicine: Washington, DC, USA, 2007.

36. Laporte, L.; Paris, J.; Guttman, H.; Russell, J.; Correa, J.A. Using a Sibling Design to Compare Childhood Adversities in Female Patients With BPD and Their Sisters. *Child Maltreat.* **2012**, *17*, 318–329.

37. Miller-Lewis, L.R.; Searle, A.K.; Sawyer, M.G.; Baghurst, P.A.; Hedley, D. Resource factors for mental health resilience in early childhood: An analysis with multiple methodologies. *Child Adolesc. Psychiatry Ment. Health* **2013**, *7*, 6.

38. Cowen, E.L.; Wyman, P.A.; Work, W.C.; Iker, M.R. A preventive intervention for enhancing resilience among highly stressed urban children. *J. Prim. Prev.* **1995**, *15*, 247–260.

39. Rutter, M. Annual Research Review: Resilience—Clinical implications: Resilience: clinical implications. *J. Child Psychol. Psychiatry* **2013**, *54*, 474–487.

40. Benson, H.; Beary, J. F.; Carol, M. P. The relaxation response. *Psychiatry* **1974**, *37*, 37–46.

41. Beary, J.F.; Benson, H. A simple psychophysiologic technique which elicits the hypometabolic changes of the relaxation response. *Psychosom. Med.* **1974**, *36*, 115–120.

42. Park, E.R.; Traeger, L.; Vranceanu, A.-M.; Scult, M.; Lerner, J.A.; Benson, H.; Denninger, J.; Fricchione, G.L. The Development of a Patient-Centered Program Based on the Relaxation Response: The Relaxation Response Resiliency Program (3RP). *Psychosomatics* **2013**, *54*, 165–174.

43. Vanderwert, R.E.; Marshall, P.J.; Nelson, C.A.; Zeanah, C.H.; Fox, N.A. Timing of Intervention Affects Brain Electrical Activity in Children Exposed to Severe Psychosocial Neglect. *PLoS ONE* **2010**, *5*, e11415.

44. Gerwin, C. Innovating in Early Head Start: Can Reducing Toxic Stress Improve Outcomes for Young Children? http://developingchild.harvard.edu/resources/stories_from_the_field/tackling_toxic_stress/innovating_in_early_head_start/ (accessed 2 May, 2014).

45. Flaherty, E.G.; Stirling, J. The Committee on Child Abuse and Neglect The Pediatrician's Role in Child Maltreatment Prevention. *PEDIATRICS* **2010**, *126*, 833–841.

46. Briggs-Gowan, M.J.; Carter, A. S. Social-Emotional Screening Status in Early Childhood Predicts Elementary School Outcomes. *PEDIATRICS* **2008**, *121*, 957–962.

47. Briggs, R.D.; Stettler, E.M.; Silver, E. J.; Schrag, R.D.A.; Nayak, M.; Chinitz, S.; Racine, A.D. Social-Emotional Screening for Infants and Toddlers in Primary Care. *PEDIATRICS* **2012**, *129*, e377–e384.

48. Title of site: http://www.aap.org/en-us/professional-resources/clinical-support/Pages/Clinical-Support.aspx (accessed 15 September, 2014).

49. Fjorback, L.O.; Arendt, M.; Ornbøl, E.; Fink, P.; Walach, H. Mindfulness-based stress reduction and mindfulness-based cognitive therapy: a systematic review of randomized controlled trials. *Acta Psychiatr. Scand.* **2011**, *124*, 102–119.

50. Lehrer, P.M.; Vaschillo, E.; Vaschillo, B.; Lu, S.-E.; Eckberg, D.L.; Edelberg, R.; Shih, W.J.; Lin, Y.; Kuusela, T.A.; Tahvanainen, K.U.O.; Hamer, R.M. Heart rate variability biofeedback increases baroreflex gain and peak expiratory flow. *Psychosom. Med.* **2003**, *65*, 796–805.

51. Smith, M.S.; Doroshow, C.; Womack, W.M.; Tenckhoff, L.; Stamm, S.; Pertik, M. Symptomatic Mitral Valve Prolapse in Children and Adolescents: Catecholamines, Anxiety, and Biofeedback. *Pediatrics* **1989**, *84*, 290–295.

52. Pasiali, V. Supporting parent-child interactions: music therapy as an intervention for promoting mutually responsive orientation. *J. Music Ther.* **2012**, *49*, 303–334.

53. Kerrigan, D.; Johnson, K.; Stewart, M.; Magyari, T.; Hutton, N.; Ellen, J. M.; Sibinga, E.M.S. Perceptions, experiences, and shifts in perspective occurring among urban youth participating in a mindfulness-based stress reduction program. *Complement. Ther. Clin. Pract.* **2011**, *17*, 96–101.

54. Sibinga, E.M.S.; Kerrigan, D.; Stewart, M.; Johnson, K.; Magyari, T.; Ellen, J.M. Mindfulness-based stress reduction for urban youth. *J. Altern. Complement. Med. N. Y. N* **2011**, *17*, 213–218.

55. Weigensberg, M.J.; Lane, C.J.; Ávila, Q.; Konersman, K.; Ventura, E.; Adam, T.; Shoar, Z.; Goran, M.I.; Spruijt-Metz, D. Imagine HEALTH: results from a randomized pilot lifestyle intervention for obese Latino adolescents using Interactive Guided ImagerySM. *BMC Complement. Altern. Med.* **2014**, *14*, 28.

56. Bothe, D.A.; Grignon, J.B.; Olness, K.N. The Effects of a Stress Management Intervention in Elementary School Children: *J. Dev. Behav. Pediatr.* **2014**, *35*, 62–67.

57. Peira, N.; Fredrikson, M.; Pourtois, G. Controlling the emotional heart: heart rate biofeedback improves cardiac control during emotional reactions. *Int. J. Psychophysiol. Off. J. Int. Organ. Psychophysiol.* **2014**, *91*, 225–231.

58. Tilt, A.C.; Werner, P.D.; Brown, D.F.; Alam, H.B.; Warshaw, A.L.; Parry, B.A.; Jazbar, B.; Booker, A.; Stangenberg, L.; Fricchione, G.L.; Benson, H.; Lillemoe, K.D.; Conrad, C. Low degree of formal education and musical experience predict degree of music-induced stress reduction in relatives and friends of patients: a single-center, randomized controlled trial. *Ann. Surg.* **2013**, *257*, 834–838.

59. Slopen, N.; McLaughlin, K.A.; Shonkoff, J. P. Interventions to Improve Cortisol Regulation in Children: A Systematic Review. *PEDIATRICS* **2014**, *133*, 312–326.

60. Shonkoff, J. P. Leveraging the biology of adversity to address the roots of disparities in health and development. *Proc. Natl. Acad. Sci. U. S. A.* **2012**, *109 Suppl 2*, 17302–17307.

61. www.helpguide.org helpguide.com (accessed 24 August, 2014).

62. www.stress.org stress.org (accessed 24 August, 2014).

63. www.heartmath heartmath.com (accessed 24 August, 2014).

64. www.heartmath.org (accessed 24 August, 2014).

65. Hoch, D.B.; Watson, A.J.; Linton, D.A.; Bello, H.E.; Senelly, M.; Milik, M.T.; Baim, M.A.; Jethwani, K.; Fricchione, G.L.; Benson, H.; Kvedar, J.C. The Feasibility and Impact of Delivering a Mind-Body Intervention in a Virtual World. *PLoS ONE* **2012**, *7*, e33843.

66. Schweinhart, L.J.; Montie, J; Xiang, Z.; Barnett, W.S.; Belfield, C.R.; Nores, M. *Lifetime effects: The HighScope Perry Preschool study through age 40*; HighScope Educational Reseach Foundation: Ypsilanti, MI, 2005.

67. Campbell, F.A.; Pungello, E.P.; Miller-Johnson, S.; Burchinal, M.; Ramey, C.T. The development of cognitive and academic abilities: growth curves from an early childhood educational experiment. *Dev. Psychol.* **2001**, *37*, 231–242.

Iron, Magnesium, Vitamin D, and Zinc Deficiencies in Children Presenting with Symptoms of Attention-Deficit/Hyperactivity Disorder

Amelia Villagomez and Ujjwal Ramtekkar

Abstract: Attention-Deficit/Hyperactivity Disorder (ADHD) is a neurodevelopmental disorder increasing in prevalence. Although there is limited evidence to support treating ADHD with mineral/vitamin supplements, research does exist showing that patients with ADHD may have reduced levels of vitamin D, zinc, ferritin, and magnesium. These nutrients have important roles in neurologic function, including involvement in neurotransmitter synthesis. The aim of this paper is to discuss the role of each of these nutrients in the brain, the possible altered levels of these nutrients in patients with ADHD, possible reasons for a differential level in children with ADHD, and safety and effect of supplementation. With this knowledge, clinicians may choose in certain patients at high risk of deficiency, to screen for possible deficiencies of magnesium, vitamin D, zinc, and iron by checking RBC-magnesium, 25-OH vitamin D, serum/plasma zinc, and ferritin. Although children with ADHD may be more likely to have lower levels of vitamin D, zinc, magnesium, and iron, it cannot be stated that these lower levels *caused* ADHD. However, supplementing areas of deficiency may be a safe and justified intervention.

Reprinted from *Children*. Cite as: Villagomez, A.; Ramtekkar, U. Iron, Magnesium, Vitamin D, and Zinc Deficiencies in Children Presenting with Symptoms of Attention-Deficit/Hyperactivity Disorder. *Children* **2014**, *1*, 261-279.

1. Introduction

Attention-deficit/hyperactivity disorder (ADHD) is a neurodevelopmental disorder characterized by impaired levels of inattention and hyperactivity in more than one setting. The rates of ADHD have risen over the past few decades and continue to rise. According to recent data from the National Survey of Children's Health, 11% of US children ages 4–17 had been diagnosed at some point in their lives with ADHD; this is a 42% increase from the 7.8% of children in 2003. By parent-report, the percentage of children aged 4–17 taking medication for ADHD was 4.8% in 2007 and 6.1% in 2011 [1].

There is no single cause of ADHD, and much research has focused on both environmental and genetic risk factors independently. Recent studies also demonstrate the complex interplay of genetic and environmental factors. For example, a genetically endowed variability of dopaminergic genotypes to specific environmental risk factors, such as prenatal smoking, can result in a specific subtype of ADHD [2]. ADHD has been associated with maternal smoking, alcohol and substance misuse, maternal stress, low birth weight and prematurity, organophosphates, polychlorinated biphenyls, lead, artificial food colorings, severe early deprivation, and family adversity. Although these factors have been correlated with ADHD and some are risk factors, none of them have been shown to definitively cause ADHD [3]. Although medications for ADHD have a large effect size and psychosocial interventions can augment treatment success, more than 30% of children are still symptomatic despite combined treatment [4].

Many parents choose not to start medication for fear of side effects and may seek "alternative" or "natural" treatments. Data from the National Health Interview Study demonstrated that for children ages 7 to 17, by parent-report, 8.9% of children had been diagnosed with ADHD, and of those, 24.7% used at least one type of complementary and alternative medical (CAM) therapy [5]. There is no conclusive data to support nutrient deficiencies as a cause of ADHD. However, research does exist demonstrating that patients with ADHD have reduced levels of vitamin D, zinc, ferritin, and magnesium. We will review the existing literature on zinc, ferritin, magnesium, and vitamin D and their association with ADHD to guide clinicians on possible appropriate laboratory screening measures for children presenting with symptoms consistent with ADHD.

2. Zinc

2.1. Role of Zinc

Zinc plays an important role for protein and DNA synthesis, in wound healing, for bone structure, and on the immune system. Deficiency of zinc can result in poor growth and retarded development, hair loss, diarrhea, suppression of aspects of cell-mediated immunity, and dermatitis. There is no pathognomonic sign for zinc deficiency and severe zinc deficiency is uncommon in the United States [6,7].

Zinc is considered a trace element because plasma concentration is only 12–16 μM; the body contains approximately 2–4 grams of zinc, the majority of which is in the bone and skeletal muscle. Only 0.1% of the total amount of zinc in the body is in the plasma [8]. The body does not store zinc, so supply must be repleted by dietary intake [9].

The Dietary Reference Intake (DRI) is the general term for a set of reference values used to plan and assess nutrient intakes of healthy individuals. The current DRI is based on the previous Recommended Daily Allowance (RDA) and is 5 mg for females and males 4–8 years old, 8 mg for females and males 9–13 years old, 9 mg for females 14–18 years old, and 11 mg for males 14–18 years old. The RDA is the amount of intake adequate for 97%–98% of the population; therefore, for 2%–3% of the population, this intake may not be sufficient [10]. In the US, meat accounts for 50% of dietary zinc intake, legumes and cereals account for 30%, and dairy products about 20% [11].

Although plant sources contain zinc, they are also high in phytic acid, which binds to zinc, forms an insoluble compound and decreases its bioavailability. According to the Institute of Medicine's report, vegetarians may require as much as a 50% greater intake of zinc given that the major source in the diet is grains and legumes which contain a high amount of phytic acid [8]. Inorganic iron and calcium supplements may decrease zinc absorption as well as alcohol, infection and surgery. Animal studies show that excessive dietary intake of calcium decreases zinc absorption, however, studies have not been done in humans.

The Tolerable Upper Intake (UL), the maximum daily intake for the general population that is unlikely to cause adverse side effects is: 12 mg for 4–7 years of age, 23 mg for 9–13 years of age, and 34 mg for 14–18 years of age. [8] There is a small window between the DRI and the UL of zinc. In adults, acute adverse side effects of excessive zinc may occur at 50–150 mg/day and include epigastric pain, nausea, loss of appetite, abdominal cramps, diarrhea and headache [8]. Chronic adverse side effects associated with excessive zinc supplementation include immune suppression, and decreased HDL cholesterol [8,12,13].

In the Health Professionals Follow-Up Study, supplemental zinc intake below 100 mg/day was not associated with increased prostate cancer risk, however men taking more than 100 mg/day had a 2.29 relative risk of advanced prostate cancer [14]. Zinc and copper compete for absorption; therefore there is a concern for copper deficiency during zinc supplementation. However, the threshold for this effect is unknown. Maret and colleagues offered the practical suggestion that until further research on this topic is done, the ratio of zinc to copper should not exceed 10–12 [7]. Sequelae of copper deficiency can include: reduced skin pigmentation, central nervous system impairment, osteoporosis, decreased immune function, anemia, and fainting spells [6].

2.2. Relevance for ADHD

Although the exact mechanism of how zinc may contribute to symptoms of ADHD is not known, it is a cofactor for more than 300 enzymes and is involved in the pathway for the body's production of prostaglandins and neurotransmitters [9]. Zinc is necessary for B6 to be metabolized to its active form, pyridoxal phosphate, which in turn plays a role in conversion of tryptophan to serotonin [15]. Zinc assists in both the production and regulation of melatonin; melatonin is an important factor in the pathophysiology of ADHD due to its modulation of dopamine [16-18]. Zinc also binds to and regulates the dopamine transporter, which is a site of action of psychostimulants used to treat ADHD [18]. However, there is no clear evidence that zinc deficiency directly results in alteration of the melatonin or dopamine transporter in children with ADHD.

There is a bidirectional association between zinc and essential fatty acids (EFAs). Zinc serves as a coenzyme of delta-6-desaturase, an enzyme crucial for EFA metabolism [19,20]. Prostaglandin E2, a product of essential fatty acid metabolism, facilitates the absorption of zinc in the gut [21]. Individuals with ADHD have been shown to have altered red blood cell fatty acid profiles, and supplementation with EFAs have been shown to have a small but significant effect for the treatment of ADHD [22-24].

2.3. Reduced Levels in ADHD

In 1981, Colquhoun and Bunday measured hair samples of 46 hyperactive children and noted that 31 had levels below the normal range; they hypothesized that zinc deficiency results in decreased levels of essential fatty acids and may contribute to hyperactivity [25]. In a Turkish study, there was a statistically lower serum zinc level in the ADHD group compared to healthy controls: 60.6 ± 9.9 µg/dL *vs.* 105.8 ± 13.2 µg/dL, respectively. Free fatty acid (FFA) levels in the ADHD group were one third of those in the control group (ADHD group: 0.176 ± 0.102 mEq/L and in control group: 0.562 ± 0.225 mEq/L with $p < 0.001$). There was a correlation between serum FFA and zinc levels. Authors postulated that the FFAs were possibly low secondary to zinc deficiency [26].

In a small study of 18 ADHD boys (ages 6–12) entering a double-blind balanced crossover comparison between one month of dextro-amphetamine and one month of placebo, there was no statistically significant difference between baseline hair zinc in ADHD *vs.* normal controls. However, higher baseline hair zinc levels predicted a greater placebo-controlled amphetamine improvement. The authors hypothesized that those with higher zinc levels had a sufficient amount of zinc for the stimulants to be effective and were not symptomatic because of zinc deficiency but rather from other causes. They further postulated that those with low levels of zinc would require zinc supplementation for an optimal stimulant response [27].

Researchers in British Columbia measured non-fasting serum zinc levels and evaluated 3-day food records on 43 children aged 6–12 with ADHD (18 taking stimulants, 9 atomoxetine, and 17 drug naïve). In this affluent sample (all but two came from homes with household income greater than $60,000), 28% and 61% aged 6–8 and 9–12 respectively did not meet the Estimated Average Requirement (EAR) for zinc. EAR is the average daily nutrient intake estimated to meet the requirements of half the healthy individuals in a particular age and gender group. The prevalence of zinc deficiency in children with ADHD in this study population was 8 times greater than the reported prevalence of zinc deficiency for normal populations (3.3% for males and 3% for females) [28]. Twenty-six percent of the children aged 6–8 and 20% of the 9–12 year olds had serum zinc levels below the 2.5th percentile of the National Health and Nutrition Examination Survey (NHANES II) cutoffs for zinc deficiency. NHANES II is a survey research program conducted by the National Center of Health Statistics (NCHS) to assess the health and nutritional status of adults and children in the United States and also forms the basis for national standards for such measurements.

A research study done in the US showed that in children with ADHD, lower serum zinc levels were associated with greater parent and teacher ratings of inattention ($r = -0.45$). However, this same correlation was not present when examining symptoms of hyperactivity/impulsivity of ADHD—there was actually a correlation in the positive direction, although insignificant and small ($r = 0.14; p = 0.35$) [29].

A Turkish study measured the event-related potentials (ERPs) for 3 groups: those with low zinc (N = 13, zinc level < 80 µg/dL) and ADHD, those with normal zinc levels (N = 14, zinc level ≥ 80 µg/dL) and ADHD, and age-matched controls without ADHD (N = 24). The plasma zinc levels were significantly lower in both ADHD groups as compared to the group without ADHD (means were 65.8 µg/dL in low zinc group and 89.5 µg/dL in zinc non-deficient group *vs.* control mean: 107.8 µg/dL). On EEG, compared to the zinc non-deficient ADHD group, the low zinc ADHD group had significantly shorter N2 latency in the frontal and parietal regions. Additionally, data demonstrated a significant positive correlation between plasma zinc levels of children with ADHD and the amplitude and latencies of N2 in the frontal region. In the context that prior work has suggested that N2 wave changes may reflect an atypical inhibition process, authors suggested that zinc deficiency may have a deleterious effect on inhibitory control in patients with ADHD [30,31].

Although not all studies have shown lower levels of zinc in children with ADHD, a systemic review looking for biomarkers for ADHD concluded that studies have found lower levels of zinc when measured in serum, plasma, urine, and hair [32]. The meta-analysis showed significantly lower levels of zinc among patients with ADHD ($d = -0.88$), however it was limited because of significant heterogeneity ($p = 0.0002$, $I^2 = 79\%$) [33].

2.4. Etiology of Lower Levels of Zinc

Zinc levels may be lower in patients with ADHD secondary to differences in dietary intake, differences in absorption, or other mechanisms [28,34]. Low zinc levels have also been associated with depression in adults [1,35]. Raison hypothesized that both Major Depressive Disorder and low zinc levels may have a common denominator: inflammation. Perhaps the drop of zinc levels is an evolutionarily acquired mechanism the body uses when trying to fight infections: less zinc means less nutrients for pathogens to utilize [3,36]. Although inconsistent, there is evidence that pro-inflammatory markers are elevated in children with ADHD [4,37]. Stress, acute trauma, and infection cause changes in hormones (e.g., cortisol) and cytokines (e.g., interleukin 6) that cause sequestration of zinc in the liver and spleen and consequently lower plasma zinc concentration [5,38,39]. Therefore, it is plausible that lower levels of zinc were seen in patients with ADHD because of an increased pro-inflammatory state.

An alternate explanation could involve increased zinc-wasting in the urine of children with ADHD. In a study by Ward and colleagues, children who were classified as "hyperactive" were given a drink with one of either 3 different types of artificial food coloring; their response was compared to children without hyperactivity. Hyperactive children ingesting the drink with sunset yellow ($n = 12$) or the tartrazine ($n = 23$) had significantly decreased levels of plasma zinc and an increase in urinary zinc as compared to controls. This led investigators to postulate that hyperactive children may be more sensitive to food coloring possibly secondary to causing zinc-wasting in urine for individuals with hyperactivity [6,7,40].

2.5. Interpreting Zinc Measurements

Only 0.1% of total body zinc is in the plasma and its concentration is tightly regulated by homeostatic mechanisms. Plasma levels may not reflect intracellular and zinc status in tissues throughout the body [8,9], and may show changes only when depletion is severe or extended [7,9,38].

A systematic review of the literature concluded that plasma zinc concentrations did respond to supplementation; however, no definitive conclusions could be made regarding its ability to change in response to marginal dietary intake [10,41]. Serum and plasma levels are virtually equivalent [11,42]. Although serum/plasma zinc are usually used as markers of zinc status in populations studies, and are accessible and convenient, there is currently no single universally accepted method to measure total body zinc status [8,43].

Frank deficiency of zinc may be detected by serum/plasma levels, but for marginal deficiency, levels may be imprecise and insensitive. Therefore, physical signs and functional affects may occur in the absence of low levels.

Additionally, independent of zinc status, plasma levels can be affected by infection, stress, low serum albumin, oral contraceptive use, steroid use, diarrhea, and phase of the menstrual cycle [8,38]. Additionally, zinc levels in the serum/plasma vary throughout the day. In a population of adult women, hour plasma zinc samples were taken, and patients were provided with standard meals at standard times. Levels decreased 30–90 min after a meal, reached the lowest point 3–4 h after the meal, increased throughout the night, and peaked in the morning before breakfast. Highest values of the day (morning) were 22% higher than lowest value at 2100 [8,44]. Various studies have used different cut offs for determining zinc deficiency. Based on NHANES data, a suggested lower cut off of serum zinc concentration of between 56 and 74 µg/dL was given (depending on fasting status and age) [8,12,13,38].

Given the limitations of measuring plasma/serum zinc alone, some researchers also measured hair and urine zinc to better ascertain zinc status in the body [14,15]. Arnold re-analyzed data from a previous double-blind, placebo-controlled crossover comparison of d–amphetamine and Efamol (evening primrose, containing 320 mg of gamma-linolenic acid per day) for treatment of ADHD to determine if there was a differential response moderated by zinc status. Gamma-linolenic acid is an omega-6 fatty acid and a precursor of the series 2 prostaglandins, which facilitates zinc absorption [7,21]. Status of zinc in the body was classified as adequate, borderline, or frank deficiency by considering levels of hair, urine, and red blood cell zinc. Hair levels were considered an indicator of long-term zinc status. Urine and red cell zinc were considered indicators of recent zinc intake. High levels of urine or hair zinc were considered either as a result of high dietary intake or excess wasting of normal intake. Efamol had greatest effect in the group that had borderline zinc status. Authors speculated that gamma-linolenic acid may have increased absorption of zinc in these patients with borderline deficiency [6,15].

2.6. Zinc as Treatment

Four studies have shown positive results for zinc in the treatment of ADHD. In Turkey, 400 boys with a mean age of 9.6 were randomized in a double blind controlled trial to zinc sulfate 150 mg (approximately 40 mg of elemental zinc) or placebo. Approximately half of subjects in both the placebo and zinc group dropped out of the trial secondary to lack of efficacy and adverse side effects. Adverse side effects were similar in the zinc and placebo group except there was a much higher incidence of children in the zinc group reporting a metallic taste in the mouth. At week 12, serum zinc levels increased as did the level of FFAs. Zinc levels increased from (88.8 ± 25.5 µg/dL) to (140.6 ± 33.6 µg/dL, $p = 0.01$) and FFA levels increased from 0.69 ± 0.39 mEq/L to 0.85 ± 0.38 mEq/L ($p = 0.03$). There was a significant improvement in hyperactivity, impulsivity, and socialization in ADHD patients; however, there was no improvement of attention. Improvement in hyperactivity, impulsivity, and social inappropriateness was more pronounced in those patients who were older, had higher BMIs, and lower pretreatment zinc and FFA values. Full therapeutic response was seen in 28.7% of the subjects in the zinc group *vs.* 20.4% in placebo group. Although the results were statistically significant, an intention-to-treat analysis was not done and dosages were in significant excess of the DRI. Authors noted that more than 70% still had significant symptoms and would likely benefit with supplementary medication [9,45].

This study was followed by a second study in Turkey, where it had been previously estimated that 20% of the children are deficient in zinc. In a double blind-randomized control trial, 226 third graders from a low socioeconomic level were studied and supplemented with 15 mg of elemental zinc syrup for 10 weeks, or a placebo. Zinc levels were drawn in a subgroup and no children were found to be deficient, however authors noted that this may have been due to an error in lab measurement. Parent rating scale showed improvement for attention deficit and hyperactivity in the zinc group but oppositional behavior deceased in the placebo group. No statistical difference in Conner's Rating Scale for Teachers was noted. When a subgroup analysis was done, in the group whose mother's education consisted of primary school or less, compared to placebo, there was a statistically significant decrease in the prevalence of children with clinically impairing levels of hyperactivity, attention deficit and oppositional behavior in study group. However, no differences were seen when examining the Conner's Rating Scale for Teachers [15,46].

In Iran, 44 outpatient children ages 5–11 with combined type ADHD and who were medication naïve, were given methylphenidate plus placebo or methylphenidate plus zinc sulfate 55 mg (elemental zinc approximately 15 mg), in a double-blind trial for 6 weeks. As assessed by the Teacher and Parent ADHD Rating Scale, symptoms improved in both groups with a significant better outcome for those in the zinc group. The treatment was tolerable with only nausea being a side effect more prevalent in the zinc group, and no one dropped out of the study b/c of side effects. However, there was a lack of a full placebo group as 13 out of 22 in the zinc group complained of having a metallic taste compared to none in the control group. Zinc levels were not measured in this study [17,18,47].

Arnold and colleagues conducted a study to determine if results could be replicated in the United States. Fifty-two children, ages 5–14, participated in a three phase trial. In phase 1, children received zinc glycinate 15 mg or placebo for 8 weeks. Phase 2 consisted of two weeks of adding open-label fixed dose d-amphetamine (AMPH) to both the double-blind zinc and placebo. Phase 3 consisted of 3 weeks of AMPH titrated to optimal clinical effect. This was followed by an open extension of 8 weeks in which participants in the placebo group were started on zinc (to allow all participants to try zinc). Although there were no significant differences in teacher or parent rating scores between the zinc and placebo group in phase 1 or 2 of the trial, data from phase three showed that the group receiving zinc 15 mg twice a day required a 37% lower dosage of AMPH when compared to placebo [18,48]. Authors speculated that this trial was unable to replicate previous response rates because prior studies were done in areas of high zinc deficiency. Zinc deficiency is more common in the Middle East (as compared to the US) due to high consumption of unleavened whole-grain bread and beans. Alternatively, differences could be attributed to the use of supplemental zinc glycinate in the US trial rather than zinc sulfate used in the Mideast trials. Given concern for possible nutrient-nutrient interaction with zinc supplementation, a safety assay was done to look at ferritin, red cell hemoglobin, and ceruloplasmin; all showed no significant changes. Dietary intake (Kids' Food Questionnaire) showed that zinc intake was at borderline minimal intake [19,20,48].

Not all studies involving zinc supplementation have produced positive results for symptoms of ADHD. In a placebo controlled trial in Guatemala, 674 children grades 1–4 in Guatemala, at risk of zinc deficiency, were randomized to zinc oxide 10 mg per day, 5 days a week *vs.* placebo for 6 months. There were no differences in mental health outcomes but serum zinc levels did increase during the study and increases were associated with decreases in internalizing symptoms but not hyperactivity or externalizing symptoms [21,49]. In a double-blind trial in Chile, 40 children with ADHD were randomized to methylphenidate + placebo *vs.* methylphenidate + zinc sulfate 10 mg/day for 6 weeks. There was no improvement in parent rating scores and a non-significant improvement in teacher's scores of the Conners Global Index. The mean zinc levels were normal at baseline, and decreased with treatment, with less decrease in zinc group, although not statistically significant: (placebo: 95.9 ± 21.5 to 77.9 ± 15.5; zinc: 90.3 ± 9.1 to 85.0 ± 12.0 µg/dL; NS) [22–24,50].

2.7. Other Considerations

One well-known side effect of psychostimulants is appetite suppression. A group of 100 children (average age of 11.2 years) with ADHD and treated with methylphenidate-ER (METH-ER) in Spain were given a food intake survey where they reported the foods they had consumed over the previous 3 days. On average, patients had been treated with METH-ER for approximately 28 months with a mean dosage of 1.02 mg/kg/day. The children with ADHD consumed an average of 1,778 calories per day and the control group consumed 2,072 calories ($p < 0.0001$). There was a statistically significant difference in zinc intake between the medicated ADHD group and the control group: 8.6 mg (SD: 2.6) of zinc *vs.* 10.2 mg/day (SD: 2.7) [25,51]. The DRI for this age group is 8 mg; therefore, a subgroup in the ADHD group was at an increased risk of zinc-deficiency secondary to poor dietary intake.

2.8. Conclusion

Zinc plays an important role in neurologic functioning. ADHD has been associated with lower levels of hair, plasma, serum, and urinary zinc. Although the efficacy of supplementation with zinc is not definitively clear, there is evidence to support that many children even in developed countries have sub-optimal levels of zinc intake. Children taking stimulants and experiencing appetite suppression may have decreased caloric intake and be at an increased risk of insufficient dietary intake of zinc. There are mixed results whether baseline zinc status predicts improvement of ADHD-related symptoms with supplementation [26,45,48]. Given that plasma zinc levels are an imprecise measurement of zinc status, normal zinc levels do not indicate adequate zinc availability to the central nervous system; however, low levels indicate deficiency in the body. Measuring more than one indicator of zinc status may provide more information regarding zinc status [15,27]. Checking plasma/serum levels of zinc (suggestive of short term zinc status) and/or hair zinc (suggestive of long term zinc status) may be appropriate for individuals not responding to conventional treatments for ADHD and populations at higher risk of zinc deficiency (e.g., vegetarians) [27,28]. It has been recommended that zinc in RDA/RDI dosages as part of a balanced vitamin/mineral supplement is a safe and cost effective intervention [29,52].

3. Magnesium

Magnesium is involved in at least 300 enzymatic reactions, and required for fatty acid synthesis. It also plays a role in muscle relaxation, protein synthesis, and energy production. Muscles contain 27% of all the magnesium in the body and bones contain 60%. Dietary sources include: whole grains, nuts, legumes, seafood, and green vegetables [6,30,31]. In animal studies, magnesium has been shown to activate tyrosine hydroxylase, the rate-limiting step in dopamine synthesis. Magnesium also binds serotonin and dopamine to their receptors [32,53].

3.1. Evidence for Differential Level

According to a study done in Poland, children with ADHD had lower levels of magnesium compared to healthy controls. Percentage of deficiency was dependent on method of measurement: 33.6% were deficient on serum magnesium, 77.6% on hair, and 58.6% on red blood cell magnesium [33,54]. In an Egyptian sample, compared to healthy controls, serum magnesium levels were lower in children with hyperactive and combined type ADHD (2.2 ± 0.9 mEq/L vs. 1.7 ± 0.8 mEq/L, $p = 0.02$); there were no differences in levels in the subgroup of children with ADHD-inattentive type. In a sample of 76 children in France, compared to healthy controls, those with ADHD had lower RBC magnesium levels. However there was not a statistical difference of serum magnesium levels between the control and ADHD group [28,34,55]. Conversely, a group of college students diagnosed with ADHD in the United States, when compared to healthy controls, had *higher* levels of serum magnesium (789.35 ± 127.22 uM vs. 630.67 ± 87.28 uM, $p = 0.002$) but when RBC magnesium levels were compared, they were no differences between groups [24]. Possible hypotheses to account for conflicting results include different dietary intake between populations and methods of magnesium assessment. Blood plasma/serum magnesium do not precisely reflect intracellular level of magnesium; this may be better reflected in RBC-mag levels [56].

3.2. Measuring Magnesium

Only 1% of magnesium is located in the extracellular space. Therefore, plasma/serum levels may not reflect intracellular levels. Furthermore, plasma/serum levels are tightly regulated; one-third of magnesium in bone is freely exchanged with the plasma; therefore, even if intake is inadequate, normal serum levels may be maintained by bone stores. A systematic review concluded that serum/plasma magnesium concentration, red blood cell concentrations (RBC-mag), and urinary magnesium are useful markers of magnesium status in healthy populations; these markers responded to changes depletion/supplementation. It is unknown whether serum/plasma magnesium or RBC-magnesium reflects intracerebral magnesium levels [56]. In clinical practice, RBC-mag is commonly used since it measures intracellular magnesium deficiency [57].

3.3. Magnesium Supplementation

A double-blind randomized controlled clinical trial has not been done to evaluate the efficacy of magnesium for ADHD. However there is preliminary evidence to suggest that magnesium may be promising to reduce the symptoms of ADHD. There are six reported studies using magnesium as an intervention for ADHD. Of these, three had a control group [58]. The largest study was an observational study of 810 children (5–12 years of age) with symptoms of inattention and behavioral problems (but not with a confirmed diagnosis of ADHD) who were supplemented with 80 mg of magnesium, zinc, eicosapentaenoic acid, docosahexaenoic acid, and gamma-linolenic acid [59]. After 12 weeks of supplementation, there was a reduction in symptoms of inattention as well as hyperactivity/impulsivity. In children with ADHD, one study showed improvement in the clinical symptoms of ADHD with a magnesium-vitamin B6 (Mg-B6) regimen (6 mg/kg/d Mg, 0.6 mg/kg/day vitamin B6), and increased RBC magnesium levels with supplementation. However, there was no statistically significant association between the increase in RBC-mag levels and degree of improvement of clinical symptoms [55].

Although magnesium supplementation normalized RBC-magnesium levels in some studies [55,60], in others, RBC magnesium levels did not normalize after supplementation although hair magnesium levels did improve [61].

Trave showed that children taking stimulants had decreased magnesium intake as compared to healthy controls (222.9 ± 49.8 mg *vs.* 291.2 ± 86.3 mg) [51]. The DRI for magnesium is 250 mg for males and females ages 9–13; therefore, some of these children may be deficient in magnesium.

3.4. Safety

Of the trials involving supplementation, only one commented on safety and adverse effects. No serious adverse effects occurred, however, 1.1% discontinued the supplement secondary to intolerance [59]. The most common adverse side effect is diarrhea; at very high dosages magnesium has caused paralytic ileus, metabolic alkalosis, and hypokalemia [62]. Based on animal studies, there is concern that in some individuals, depending on dosage, supplementation may cause increase in aggression [52,53]. It has been suggested that moderate doses (up to 200 mg/day) pass the criteria of being a safe, inexpensive, and possibly efficacious adjunctive treatment for individuals with ADHD [52].

3.5. Summary

There is preliminary evidence to suggest that a subgroup of patients presenting with hyperactivity, impulsivity, and inattention may be deficient in magnesium. It is unclear if this is true for only certain regions of the world. Some individuals may be at higher risk for magnesium deficiency (e.g. those with appetite suppression or proton pump inhibitors [63]). In individuals presenting with symptoms of AHD, where there is clinical suspicion for magnesium deficiency, clinicians may consider measuring RBC-mag levels.

4. Vitamin D

4.1. Basic Functions, Sources, and Relevance for ADHD

In addition to its regulation of calcium and phosphorous in the intestine and stimulation of bone cell mineralization, vitamin D is a neuroactive steroid that has been shown in both animal and human studies to be important for normal brain development [6,64]. Vitamin D receptors and 1α-hydroxylase enzyme (1α-OHase), an enzyme responsible for the formation of the active form of vitamin D, are located throughout the central nervous system. Vitamin D receptors and enzymes are located in neuronal cells of the substantia nigra, hippocampus, hypothalamus, prefrontal cortex, and cingulated gyrus; many of these regions have also been shown to have abnormalities in ADHD [65,66]. There is data to suggest that Vitamin D deficiency during development has deleterious effects on the dopamine system and, in animal models, vitamin D has been shown to be associated with the production of tyrosine hydroxylase, the rate-limiting enzyme for dopamine synthesis [67,68]. Vitamin D may exert its neurological effects through various mechanisms. In animal models, it has been shown that vitamin D is an important factor for the differentiation of developing brain cells, is involved in axonal growth, can increase antioxidants such as glutathione and therefore protect against oxidative stress, and can regulate various neurotrophic factors such as nerve growth factor. Although largely cross-sectional in design, there have been studies demonstrating an association between low vitamin D levels with schizophrenia, depression, and Alzheimer's Disease [68].

4.2. Measuring Vitamin D

Although 1,25-dihydroxyvitamin D is the active form of vitamin D, serum levels are not considered a useful measure of vitamin D status in the body because its half-life is short and it may remain normal even in deficiency secondary to up-regulation of the 1α-OHase enzyme. 25-hydroxyvitamin D (25-OH) is agreed to be the best measure of Vitamin D and reflects both cutaneous synthesis and intake from food and supplements. Although there is debate in the literature regarding optimal levels of Vitamin D, individuals with 25-hydroxyvitamin D levels below 20 ng/mL (50 nmol/L) are considered deficient and levels above 50 ng/mL (125 nmol/L) may cause potential adverse effects. For vitamin D, the current Recommended Dietary Allowance is based on data for bone health. The Institute of Medicine determined in their 2011 report that there was insufficient evidence to show a causal relationship between vitamin D and extraskeletal outcomes. The Recommended Dietary Allowance for individuals ages 1–70 is 600 IU/day. The tolerable upper intake levels for children ages 4–8 is 3,000 IU/day and for children 9 and above is 4,000 IU/day [69].

4.3. Sources

Provitamin D molecules in the skin are converted by sunlight to vitamin D. Dietary sources of vitamin D include fatty fish, eggs, butter, liver, and fortified foods like milk [6]. Individuals at increased risk for insufficient amounts of vitamin D include those with darker skin pigmentation, limited sun exposure, kidney disease, liver disease, disorders of malabsorption, and taking some antiepileptic drugs [70].

4.4. Evidence for Differential Level

In a case control study done in Qatar, 1,331 children diagnosed with ADHD (ages 5–18) based on clinical diagnosis and rating scales, were matched with children without ADHD. There was a statistically lower level of 25-OH vitamin D (16.6 ± 7.8 ng/mL) in the ADHD group compared with healthy controls (23.5 ± 9.0 ng/mL, $p < 0.001$). These correlations continued to be true after adjusting for BMI and gender (adj. OR = 1.54 with CI of 1.32–1.81, $p < 0.001$). 19.1% of children with ADHD *vs.* 12.7% of healthy controls had 25-OH vitamin D levels of less than 10 ng/mL, indicating severe deficiency. Limitations of the study included that dietary intake was not measured nor amount of time in the sun; therefore, it is unclear if these changes were due to differences in the amount of sunlight exposure, dietary intake, or metabolism of vitamin D. Even in sun-rich countries, vitamin D deficiency exists in part due to limited time outdoors because of extreme climates [71].

In a cross section study, a group in Turkey measured 25-OH vitamin D in children (ages 9 ± 2.2 years old) diagnosed with ADHD ($n = 60$) and compared these to a healthy control group (10.1 ± 3.3 years old). The ADHD group had statistically lower levels of 25-OH vitamin D (20.9 ± 19.4 *vs.* 34.9 ± 15.4 ng/mL). No differences were noted in levels of calcium, phosphorous, or alkaline phosphatase and levels of vitamin D were not different in the three subgroups (inattentive *vs.* hyperactive/impulsive *vs.* combined) [72].

4.5. Summary

There are no current studies in children using vitamin D as a treatment for ADHD, but two studies show lower levels of vitamin D in individuals with ADHD. There are vitamin D receptors in key areas of the brain implicated in ADHD, and increasing research showing the importance of this vitamin in brain development. Clinicians may consider measuring 25-OH vitamin D levels in some individuals with symptoms of ADHD, especially in those with other risk factors.

5. Iron

A systemic review of the literature examining the association of iron and ADHD was recently published; the reader is referred to this article for a more comprehensive review [73]. Iron is necessary for the synthesis of catecholames and dopamine. Ferritin is a marker of peripheral iron stores, and can be used to estimate body-iron stores; however, it is not known if it reflects brain iron [73]. Although some studies have shown lower levels of ferritin in children with ADHD, other studies have not found this correlation; therefore, current results are mixed [73–75]. There is only one randomized-placebo controlled trial ($n = 23$) evaluating the efficacy of ferrous sulfate (80 mg) for non-anemic children with ADHD and low ferritin levels (<30 ng/mL); supplementation showed some improvement of symptoms of ADHD [76].

Studies have estimated the prevalence of Restless Leg Symptoms (RLS)/RLS symptoms in patients with ADHD to be up to 44% [77]. In 2003, a report from a National Institutes of Health (NIH) consensus conference defined four essential criteria of RLS: urge to move the legs, worse with rest/inactivity, worse in the evening, and relieved by movement. For children, there is an additional criteria of the child expressing leg discomfort in their own words [78]. It is hypothesized that a common dysfunction of the dopamine system accounts for the high comorbidity. There is currently no definitive treatment algorithm for children presenting with RLS [79]. In children with RLS and low ferritin (less than 40 ng/mL), iron supplementation was found to be effective for improving symptoms of ADHD in a small open-label study [80]. Given the high comorbidity, children with symptoms of ADHD should be screened for RLS, and in those with RLS, measuring serum ferritin should be considered.

6. Conclusions

Many symptoms of ADHD are addressed with behavioral therapy and medications; however, even with combined treatments, one-third of patients are still symptomatic [4]. Currently there is no evidence to support supplementation as a monotherapy for the treatment of ADHD, however, supplementation may improve medication response and overall well-being, especially in those with deficiencies. Although it is not definitively clear the percentage of children presenting with symptoms of ADHD who have nutrient deficiencies, the existing literature suggests that a subgroup of children with ADHD are at risk for nutrient deficiencies which may play a role in symptomology. In children presenting symptoms of ADHD, clinicians are encouraged to review the dietary history, consider risk factors for zinc, iron, magnesium, and vitamin D deficiency and order RBC-magnesium, 25-OH vitamin D, ferritin, and serum zinc when appropriate (see Table 1).

Key acronyms: 25-OH (25-hydroxyvitamin D), RDA (Recommended Daily Allowance), DRI (Dietary reference intake), UL (Tolerable Upper Intake), EFA (Essential fatty acids), EAR (Estimated average requirement).

Table 1. Possible Nutrient Deficiencies in Children with ADHD

Nutrient	Existing Evidence for Differential Levels in Children with ADHD	Children at Additional Risk for Nutrient Deficiency	Laboratory Measurement
Zinc	Yes	vegetarians, poor dietary intake of zinc-rich foods	Serum/plasma zinc and/or hair zinc
Magnesium	Yes	poor dietary intake of magnesium-rich foods (whole grains, nuts, legumes, seafood, green vegetables), consuming medications that decrease magnesium absorption (e.g. proton pump inhibitors)	RBC-magnesium
Vitamin D	Yes	darker skin pigmentation, limited sun exposure, kidney disease, liver disease, disorders of malabsorption	25-OH Vitamin D
Iron	Yes	poor dietary intake of iron	Ferritin

Acknowledgments

Support was received from the University of Arizona Strategic Priorities Faculty Initiative.

Author Contributions

A.V. prepared the manuscript for the sections on magnesium, ferritin, and zinc. U.R. assisted in the conceptualization, editing, and section on ferritin.

Conflicts of Interest

The authors declare no conflict of interest.

References

1. Visser, S.N.; Danielson, M.L.; Bitsko, R.H.; Holbrook, J.R.; Kogan, M.D.; Ghandour, R.M.; Perou, R.; Blumberg, S.J. Trends in the Parent-Report of Health Care Provider-Diagnosed and Medicated Attention-Deficit/Hyperactivity Disorder: United States, 2003–2011. *J. Am. Acad. Child Adolesc. Psychiatry* **2014**, *53*, 34–46.e2.
2. Neuman, R.J.; Lobos, E.; Reich, W.; Henderson, C.A.; Sun, L.-W.; Todd, R.D. Prenatal smoking exposure and dopaminergic genotypes interact to cause a severe ADHD subtype. *Biol. Psychiatry* **2007**, *61*, 1320–1328.
3. Thapar, A.; Cooper, M.; Eyre, O.; Langley, K. Practitioner Review: What have we learnt about the causes of ADHD? *J. Child Psychol. Psychiatry* **2012**, *54*, 3–16.
4. Swanson, J.M.; Kraemer, H.C.; Hinshaw, S.P.; Arnold, L.E.; Conners, C.K.; Abikoff, H.B.; Clevenger, W.; Davies, M.; Elliott, G.R.; Greenhill, L.L.; *et al.* Clinical relevance of the primary findings of the MTA: success rates based on severity of ADHD and ODD symptoms at the end of treatment. *J. Am. Acad. Child Adolesc. Psychiatry* **2001**, *40*, 168–179.
5. Kemper, K.J.; Gardiner, P.; Birdee, G.S. Use of Complementary and Alternative Medical Therapies Among Youth With Mental Health Concerns. *Acad. Pediatr.* **2013**, *13*, 540–545.
6. Liska, D.; Quinn, S.; Lukaczer, D.; Jones, D.; Lerman, R. *Textbook of Clinical Nutrition: A Functional Approach*, 2nd ed; The Institute for Functional Medicine: Gig Harbor, Washington, DC, USA, 2004; pp. 171–172.
7. Maret, W.; Sandstead, H.H. Zinc requirements and the risks and benefits of zinc supplementation. *J. Trace Elem. Med. Biol.* **2006**, *20*, 3–18.
8. Institute of Medicine (U.S.). *Panel on Micronutrients DRI: Dietary Reference Intakes for Vitamin A, Vitamin K, Arsenic, Boron, Chromium, Copper, Iodine, Iron, Manganese, Molybdenum, Nickel, Silicon, Vanadium, and Zinc:* A Report of the Panel on Micronutrients and the Standing Committee on the Scientific Evaluation of Dietary Reference Intakes, Food and Nutrition Board, Institute of Medicine; National Academy Press: Washington, DC, USA, 2001.
9. Rink, L.; Gabriel, P. Zinc and the immune system. *Proc. Nutr. Soc.* **2000**, *59*, 541–552.

10. U.S. Department of Agriculture and U.S. Department of Health and Human Services. *Dietary Guidelines for Americans, 2010.* 7th ed., Government Printing Office: Washington, DC, USA.

11. Walsh, C.T.; Sandstead, H.H.; Prasad, A.S.; Newberne, P.M.; Fraker, P.J. Zinc: Health effects and research priorities for the 1990s. *Environ. Health Perspect.* **1994**, *102* (*Suppl. 2*), 5–46.

12. Chandra, R.K. Excessive intake of zinc impairs immune responses. *JAMA* **1984**, *252*, 1443–1446.

13. Porea, T.J.; Belmont, J.W.; Mahoney, D.H., Jr. Zinc-induced anemia and neutropenia in an adolescent. *J. Pediatr.* **2000**, *136*, 688–690.

14. Leitzmann, M.F.; Stampfer, M.J.; Wu, K.; Colditz, G.A.; Willett, W.C.; Giovannucci, E.L. Zinc supplement use and risk of prostate cancer. *J. Natl. Cancer Inst.* **2003**, *95*, 1004–1007.

15. Arnold, L.E.; Pinkham, S.M.; Votolato, N. Does zinc moderate essential fatty acid and amphetamine treatment of attention-deficit/hyperactivity disorder? *J. Child Adolesc. Psychopharmacol.* **2000**, *10*, 111–117.

16. Kirby, K.; Floriani, V.; Bernstein, H. Diagnosis and management of attention-deficit/hyperactivity disorder in children. *Curr. Opin. Pediatr.* **2001**, *13*, 190–199.

17. Chen, M.D.; Lin, P.Y.; Sheu, W.H. Zinc coadministration attenuates melatonin's effect on nitric oxide production in mice. *Biol. Trace Elem. Res.* **1999**, *69*, 261–268.

18. Lepping, P.; Huber, M. Role of Zinc in the Pathogenesis of Attention-Deficit Hyperactivity Disorder. *CNS Drugs* **2010**, *24*, 721–728.

19. Bettger, W.J.; Reeves, P.G.; Moscatelli, E.A.; Reynolds, G.; O'Dell, B.L. Interaction of zinc and essential fatty acids in the rat. *J. Nutr.* **1979**, *109*, 480–488.

20. Arnold, L.E.; Disilvestro, R.A. Zinc in attention-deficit/hyperactivity disorder. *J. Child. Adolesc. Psychopharmacol.* **2005**, *15*, 619–627.

21. Song, M.K.; Adham, N.F. Evidence for an important role of prostaglandins E2 and F2 in the regulation of zinc transport in the rat. *J. Nutr.* **1979**, *109*, 2152–2159.

22. Arnold, L.E. Fish Oil Is Not Snake Oil. *J. Am. Acad. Child Adolesc. Psychiatry* **2011**, *50*, 969–971.

23. Bloch, M.H.; Qawasmi, A. Omega-3 Fatty Acid Supplementation forthe Treatment of Children With Attention-Deficit/Hyperactivity DisorderSymptomatology: Systematic Review andMeta-Analysis. *J. Am. Acad. Child Adolesc. Psychiatry* **2011**, *50*, 991–1000.

24. Antalis, C.J.; Stevens, L.J.; Campbell, M.; Pazdro, R.; Ericson, K.; Burgess, J.R. Omega-3 fatty acid status in attention-deficit/hyperactivity disorder. *Prostaglandins Leukot. Essent. Fatty Acids* **2006**, *75*, 299–308.

25. Colquhoun, I.; Bunday, S. A lack of essential fatty acids as a possible cause of hyperactivity in children. *Med. Hypotheses* **1981**, *7*, 673–679.

26. Bekaroğlu, M.; Aslan, Y.; Gedik, Y.; Değer, O.; Mocan, H.; Erduran, E.; Karahan, C. Relationships between serum free fatty acids and zinc, and attention deficit hyperactivity disorder: A research note. *J. Child Psychol. Psychiatry* **1996**, *37*, 225–227.

27. Arnold, L.E.; Votolato, N.A.; Kleykamp, D.; Baker, G.B.; Bornstein, R.A. Does hair zinc predict amphetamine improvement of ADD/hyperactivity? *Int. J. Neurosci.* **1990**, *50*, 103–107.

28. Kiddie, J.Y.; Weiss, M.D.; Kitts, D.D.; Levy-Milne, R.; Wasdell, M.B. Nutritional Status of Children with Attention Deficit Hyperactivity Disorder: A Pilot Study. *Int. J. Pediatr.* **2010**, doi:10.1155/2010/767318.

29. Arnold, L.E.; Bozzolo, H.; Hollway, J.; Cook, A.; Disilvestro, R.A.; Bozzolo, D.R.; Crowl, L.; Ramadan, Y.; Williams, C. Serum zinc correlates with parent- and teacher- rated inattention in children with attention-deficit/hyperactivity disorder. *J. Child. Adolesc. Psychopharmacol.* **2005**, *15*, 628–636.

30. Yorbik, O.; Ozdag, M.F.; Olgun, A.; Senol, M.G.; Bek, S.; Akman, S. Potential effects of zinc on information processing in boys with attention deficit hyperactivity disorder. *Prog. Neuropsychopharmacol. Biol. Psychiatry* **2008**, *32*, 662–667.

31. Barry, R.J.; Johnstone, S.J.; Clarke, A.R. A review of electrophysiology in attention-deficit/hyperactivity disorder: II. Event-related potentials. *Clin. Neurophysiol.* **2003**, *114*, 184–198.

32. McGee, R.; Williams, S.; Anderson, J.; McKenzie-Parnell, J.M.; Silva, P.A. Hyperactivity and serum and hair zinc levels in 11-year-old children from the general population. *Biol. Psychiatry* **1990**, *28*, 165–168.

33. Scassellati, C.; Bonvicini, C.; Faraone, S.V.; Gennarelli, M. Review: Biomarkers and Attention-Deficit/Hyperactivity Disorder: A Systematic Review and Meta-Analyses. *J. Am. Acad. Child Adolesc. Psychiatry* **2012**, *51*, 1003–1019.e20.

34. Stevens, L.J.; Zentall, S.S.; Deck, J.L.; Abate, M.L.; Watkins, B.A.; Lipp, S.R.; Burgess, J.R. Essential fatty acid metabolism in boys with attention-deficit hyperactivity disorder. *Am. J. Clin. Nutr.* **1995**, *62*, 761–768.

35. Swardfager, W.; Herrmann, N.; Mazereeuw, G.; Goldberger, K.; Harimoto, T.; Lanctôt, K.L. Zinc in Depression: A Meta-Analysis. *Biol. Psychiatry* **2013**, *74*, 872–878.

36. Raison, C. Depression, Zinc, and an Evolutionary Arms Race; Psych Congress Network. Available online: http://www.psychcongress.com/blogs/charles-raison-md/depression-zinc-and-evolutionary-arms-race (accessed on 11 May 2014).

37. Mitchell, R.; Goldstein, B. REVIEW: Inflammation in Children and Adolescents With Neuropsychiatric Disorders: A Systematic Review. *J. Am. Acad. Child Adolesc. Psychiatry* **2014**, *53*, 274–296.

38. Hotz, C.; Peerson, J.M.; Brown, K.H. Suggested lower cutoffs of serum zinc concentrations for assessing zinc status: Reanalysis of the second National Health and Nutrition Examination Survey data (1976–1980). *Am. J. Clin. Nutr.* **2003**, *78*, 756–764.

39. Thompson, R.P. Assessment of zinc status. *Proc. Nutr. Soc.* **1991**, *50*, 19–28.

40. Ward, N.I. Assessment of Chemical Factors in Relation to Child Hyperactivity. *J. Nutr. Environ. Med.* **1997**, *7*, 333–342.

41. Lowe, N.M.; Fekete, K.; Decsi, T. Methods of assessment of zinc status in humans: A systematic review. *Am. J. Clin. Nutr.* **2009**, *89*, 2040S–2051S.

42. English, J.L.; Hambidge, K. Plasma and serum zinc concentrations: Effect of time between collection and separation. *Clin. Chim. Acta* **1988**, *175*, 211–215.

43. Wood, R.J. Assessment of marginal zinc status in humans. *J. Nutr.* **2000**, *130*, 1350S–1354S.

44. Hambidge, K.M.; Goodall, M.J.; Stall, C.; Pritts, J. Post-prandial and daily changes in plasma zinc. *J. Trace Elem. Electrolytes Health Dis.* **1989**, *3*, 55–57.
45. Bilici, M.; Yıldırım, F.; Kandil, S.; Bekaroğlu, M.; Yıldırmış, S.; Değer, O.; Ülgen, M.; Yıldıran, A.; Aksu, H. Double-blind, placebo-controlled study of zinc sulfate in the treatment of attention deficit hyperactivity disorder. *Prog. Neuropsychopharmacol. Biol. Psychiatry* **2004**, *28*, 181–190.
46. Üçkardeş, Y.; Özmert, E.N.; Ünal, F.; Yurdakök, K. Effects of zinc supplementation on parent and teacher behaviour rating scores in low socioeconomic level Turkish primary school children. *Acta Paediatrica* **2009**, *98*, 731–736.
47. Akhondzadeh, S.; Mohammadi, M.-R.; Khademi, M. Zinc sulfate as an adjunct to methylphenidate for the treatment of attention deficit hyperactivity disorder in children: A double blind and randomized trial. *BMC Psychiatry* **2004**, *4*, 9.
48. Arnold, L.E.; Disilvestro, R.A.; Bozzolo, D.; Bozzolo, H.; Crowl, L.; Fernandez, S.; Ramadan, Y.; Thompson, S.; Mo, X.; Abdel-Rasoul, M.; Joseph, E. Zinc for attention-deficit/hyperactivity disorder: Placebo-controlled double-blind pilot trial alone and combined with amphetamine. *J. Child. Adolesc. Psychopharmacol.* **2011**, *21*, 1–19.
49. DiGirolamo, A.M.; Ramirez-Zea, M. Role of zinc in maternal and child mental health. *Am. J. Clin. Nutr.* **2009**, *89*, 940S–945S.
50. Zamora, J.; Velásquez, A.; Troncoso, L.; Barra, P.; Guajardo, K.; Castillo-Duran, C. Zinc en la terapia del síndrome de déficit de atención e hiperactividad en niños. Un estudio controlado aleatorio preliminar. *Arch. Latinoam. Nutr.* **2011**, *61*, 242–246.
51. Durá Travé, T.; Diez Bayona, V.; Yoldi Petri, M.E.; Aguilera Albesa, S. Dietary patterns in patients with attention deficit hyperactivity disorder. *Anal. Pediatr.* **2014**, *80*, 206–213.
52. Arnold, L.E.; Hurt, E.; Lofthouse, N. Attention-Deficit/Hyperactivity Disorder: Dietary and Nutritional Treatments. *Child Adolesc. Psychiatry Clin. NA* **2013**, *22*, 381–402.
53. Izenwasser, S.E.; Garcia-Valdez, K.; Kantak, K.M. Stimulant-like effects of magnesium on aggression in mice. *Pharmacol. Biochem. Behav.* **1986**, *25*, 1195–1199.
54. Kozielec, T.; Starobrat-Hermelin, B. Assessment of magnesium levels in children with attention deficit hyperactivity disorder (ADHD). *Magn. Res.* **1997**, *10*, 143–148.
55. Mousain-Bosc, M.; Roche, M.; Polge, A.; Pradal-Prat, D.; Rapin, J.; Bali, J.P. Improvement of neurobehavioral disorders in children supplemented with magnesium-vitamin B6. I. Attention deficit hyperactivity disorders. *Magn. Res.* **2006**, *19*, 46–52.
56. Witkowski, M.; Hubert, J.; Mazur, A. Methods of assessment of magnesium status in humans: A systematic review. *Magn. Res.* **2011**, *24*, 163–180.
57. Millart, H.; Durlach, V; Durlach, J. Red blood cell magnesium concentrations: Analytical problems and significance. *Magn. Res.* **1995**, *8*, 65–76.
58. Ghanizadeh, A. A systematic review of magnesium therapy for treating attention deficit hyperactivity disorder. *Arch. Iran. Med. (AIM)* **2013**, *16*, 412–417.

59. Huss, M.; Völp, A.; Stauss-Grabo, M. Supplementation of polyunsaturated fatty acids, magnesium and zinc in children seeking medical advice for attention-deficit/hyperactivity problems—An observational cohort study. *Lipids Health Dis.* **2010**, *9*, 105, doi:10.1186/1476-511X-9-105.

60. Mousain-Bosc, M.; Roche, M.; Rapin, J.; Bali, J.-P. Magnesium VitB6 intake reduces central nervous system hyperexcitability in children. *J. Am. Coll. Nutr.* **2004**, *23*, 545S–548S.

61. Starobrat-Hermelin, B.; Kozielec, T. The effects of magnesium physiological supplementation on hyperactivity in children with attention deficit hyperactivity disorder (ADHD). Positive response to magnesium oral loading test. *Magn. Res.* **1997**, *10*, 149–156.

62. Institute of Medicine (US) Standing Committee on the Scientific Evaluation of Dietary Reference Intakes. *Dietary Reference Intakes for Calcium, Phosphorus, Magnesium, Vitamin D, and Fluoride*; National Academies Press: Washington, DC, USA, 1997.

63. Markovits, N.; Loebstein, R.; Halkin, H.; Bialik, M.; Landes-Westerman, J.; Lomnicky, J.; Kurnik, D. The association of proton pump inhibitors and hypomagnesemia in the community setting. *J. Clin. Pharmacol.* **2014**, *54*, 889–895.

64. Harms, L.R.; Eyles, D.W.; McGrath, J.J.; Mackay-Sim, A.; Burne, T.H.J. Developmental vitamin D deficiency alters adult behaviour in 129/SvJ and C57BL/6J mice. *Behav. Brain Res.* **2008**, *187*, 343–350.

65. Eyles, D.W.; Smith, S.; Kinobe, R.; Hewison, M.; McGrath, J.J. Distribution of the Vitamin D receptor and 1α-hydroxylase in human brain. *J. Chem. Neuroanat.* **2005**, *29*, 21–30.

66. Ellison-Wright, I.; Ellison-Wright, Z.; Bullmore, E. Structural brain change in Attention Deficit Hyperactivity Disorder identified by meta-analysis. *BMC Psychiatry* **2008**, *8*, 51.

67. Sanchez, B.; Relova, J.L.; Gallego, R.; Ben-Batalla, I.; Perez-Fernandez, R. 1,25-Dihydroxyvitamin D3 administration to 6-hydroxydopamine-lesioned rats increases glial cell line-derived neurotrophic factor and partially restores tyrosine hydroxylase expression in substantia nigra and striatum. *J. Neurosci. Res.* **2009**, *87*, 723–732.

68. Eyles, D.W.; Burne, T.H.J.; McGrath, J.J. Frontiers in Neuroendocrinology. *Front. Neuroendocrinol.* **2013**, *34*, 47–64.

69. Institute of Medicine (US) Committee to Review Dietary Reference Intakes for Vitamin D and Calcium; Ross, A.C.; Taylor, C.L.; Yaktine, A.L.; del Valle, H.B. *Dietary Reference Intakes for Calcium and Vitamin D*; National Academies Press: Washington, DC, USA, 2011.

70. Kennel, K.A.; Drake, M.T.; Hurley, D.L. Vitamin D Deficiency in Adults: When to Test and How to Treat. *Mayo Clin. Proc.* **2010**, *85*, 752–758.

71. Kamal, M.; Bener, A.; Ehlayel, M.S. Is high prevalence of vitamin D deficiency a correlate for attention deficit hyperactivity disorder? *Atten. Defic. Hyperact Disord.* **2014**, *6*, 73–78.

72. Goksugur, S.B.; Tufan, A.E.; Semiz, M.; Gunes, C.; Bekdas, M.; Tosun, M.; Demircioglu, F. Vitamin D Status in Children with Attention Deficit Hyperactivity Disorder. *Pediatr. Int.* **2014**, doi:10.1111/ped.12286.

73. Cortese, S.; Angriman, M.; Lecendreux, M.; Konofal, E. Iron and attention deficit/hyperactivity disorder: What is the empirical evidence so far? A systematic review of the literature. *Expert Rev. Neurother.* **2012**, *12*, 1227–1240.

74. Oner, P.; Dirik, E.B.; Taner, Y.; Caykoylu, A.; Anlar, O. Association between low serum ferritin and restless legs syndrome in patients with attention deficit hyperactivity disorder. *Tohoku J. Exp. Med.* **2007**, *213*, 269–276.

75. Mahmoud, M.M.; El-Mazary, A.-A.M.; Maher, R.M.; Saber, M.M. Zinc, ferritin, magnesium and copper in a group of Egyptian children with attention deficithyperactivity disorder. *Ital. J. Pediatr.* **2011**, *37*, 60, doi:10.1186/1824-7288-37-60.

76. Konofal, E.; Lecendreux, M.; Deron, J.; Marchand, M.; Cortese, S.; Zaïm, M.; Mouren, M.C.; Arnulf, I. Effects of Iron Supplementation on Attention Deficit Hyperactivity Disorder in Children. *Pediatr. Neurol.* **2008**, *38*, 20–26.

77. Cortese, S.; Konofal, E.; Lecendreux, M.; Arnulf, I.; Mouren, M.C.; Darra, F.; Dalla Bernardina, B. Restless legs syndrome and attention-deficit/hyperactivity disorder: A review of the literature. *Sleep* **2005**, *28*, 1007–1013.

78. Allen, R.P.; Picchietti, D.; Hening, W.A.; Trenkwalder, C.; Walters, A.S.; Montplaisi, J. Restless legs syndrome: Diagnostic criteria, special considerations, and epidemiology. *Sleep Med.* **2003**, *4*, 101–119.

79. Blum, N.J.; Mason, T.B.A. Restless Legs Syndrome: What Is a Pediatrician to Do? *Pediatrics* **2007**, *120*, 438–439.

80. Furudate, N.; Komada, Y.; Kobayashi, M.; Nakajima, S.; Inoue, Y. Journal of the Neurological Sciences. *J. Neurol. Sci.* **2014**, *336*, 232–236.

Vitamin D in Children's Health

Joy A. Weydert

Abstract: Knowledge of vitamin D in the health of children has grown greatly over the years, extending past the importance for calcium homeostasis and bone growth. There is growing recognition of the role vitamin D plays in health impacting the innate immune system to prevent infections and the adaptive immune system to modulate autoimmunity. Other studies are starting to reveal the neurohormonal effects of vitamin D on brain development and behavior, with a link to mental health disorders. Many of these effects start well before the birth of the child, so it is important that each pregnant woman be assessed for vitamin D deficiency and supplemented for the best possible health outcome of the child. It is recommended that targeting a 25(OH)D level of 40–70 ng/mL for each individual would provide optimal health benefits and reduce health care costs. Current recommended doses of vitamin D supplementation fall short of what is needed to obtain ideal serum levels. A vitamin D supplementation program to prevent disease, much like the current vaccination program, could potentially have a dramatic impact on overall health worldwide.

Reprinted from *Children*. Cite as: Weydert, J.A. Vitamin D in Children's Health. *Children* **2014**, *1*, 208-226.

1. Introduction

The role of vitamin D has been widely publicized in the popular press promoting health benefits beyond that of bone mineralization. Some of the claims state that vitamin D reduces the incidence of cancer, prevents viral illnesses, treats musculoskeletal pain and stabilizes mood disorders such as depression. There has also been increased interest in the scientific community to study vitamin D both at the basic science and clinical levels to address these claims plus others. From Pub Med [1] greater than 60,000 citations are available related to vitamin D alone. As a result, a wealth of information has been produced that adds to our understanding of how this hormone affects virtually every cell in the body.

In this article, basic vitamin D biochemistry will be reviewed to present the current understanding of its action on various systems throughout the body. Additionally, literature from basic science and clinical studies on vitamin D in relation to current disease states will be presented. Lastly, there will be a discussion on the potential economic impact on health care if Vitamin D levels were optimized for all individuals starting before birth.

2. Discussion

2.1. Vitamin D Biochemistry

In contrast to its name, vitamin D is not a vitamin, but rather a steroid hormone. Vitamins are anti-oxidants or co-factors in enzymatic reaction that primarily come from food. Steroid hormones, on the other hand, regulate gene expression—turning on and off protein production as the body requires. Vitamin D is produced by activation of plant and animal sterol fractions, phytosterol and cholesterol respectively, by sunlight (Figure 1). Plant sterols activated by UVB irradiation produce vitamin D-2. In animals and humans, 7-dehydrocholesterol, the vitamin D precursor found primarily in the epidermal layer of the skin, is activated by sunlight to produce vitamin D-3 and is bound to vitamin D binding protein (VBP). This is transported to the liver where it is rapidly hydroxylated by vitamin D-25-hydroxylase to form 25-hydroxyvitamin D [25(OH)D], the major circulating form of vitamin D. This is considered a pro-hormone with no innate hormone activity in this state [2]. Through further hydroxylation by the enzyme 25-hydroxyvitamin D-1-α-hydroxylase, 25 (OH)D is converted into the biologically active form, 1,25 di-hydroxyvitamin D [1,25(OH)$_2$D]. 1,25 di-hydroxyvitamin D regulates more than 200 different genes, directly or indirectly, by binding to vitamin D nuclear hormone receptors (VDR) that drive a wide variety of biological processes. Most of the conversion of 25 (OH)D to 1,25(OH)$_2$D occurs in the kidney and is tightly regulated by parathyroid hormone (PTH), calcium, and phosphorus levels. In this activated state, vitamin D has classic endocrine effects and regulates serum calcium and bone metabolism [3]. The conversion to 1,25(OH)$_2$D also occurs in various tissues such as brain, breast, and skin, and in monocytes and macrophages. This local production of 1,25(OH)$_2$D regulates cell proliferation, differentiation, and apoptosis as well as augment immune function at those sites [4]. Through this mechanism, vitamin D affects cells directly by its autocrine and paracrine functions and is under autonomous control [5]. VDR are found ubiquitously in the nucleus of all tissues and cells of the immune system and can respond to the activated 1,25(OH)$_2$D for gene expression at virtually any site in the body. Having these various endocrine and paracrine functions may explain why vitamin D has wide spread effects on various disease processes.

Having adequate levels of 25 (OH)D is crucial for optimal production of activated 1,25(OH)$_2$D. Food provides a limited source of Vitamin D (salmon, sardines, tuna, cod-liver oil for Vitamin D3, and egg yolks or shiitake mushrooms for Vitamin D2) therefore diet alone only provides 100 to 200 IU of vitamin D per day. Exposure to sunlight, in contrast, produces 10,000 to 20,000 IU when 30% of the body surface area is exposed to sunlight 15 to 30 min a day [6]. Sunlight produces UVA, UVB, and UVC rays, each with different skin penetrations and biological actions. It is only a very narrow band of UVB rays (290–320 nm) that activates the 7-dehydrocholesterol in the epidermis. The UVB rays that reach the earth's surface is directly affected by the zenith angle of the sun. Very little UVB reaches the earth's surface in the early morning or late afternoon hours of the day due to the oblique nature of the sun's rays. UVB rays that are most efficient in producing vitamin D are available when the sun is most perpendicular to the earth's surface—between 10 AM and 3 PM. The zenith angle is also affected by season and latitude. In the northern and southern hemispheres, beyond the 33° latitude, the zenith angle is at its minimum during the winter months with virtually no vitamin D production possible [7].

Besides season, time of day, and latitude, UVB exposure is limited by other factors. Sunscreens reduce vitamin D production by 95% (SPF 8) to 99% (SPF 15). Institutionalized persons in prisons, schools, nursing homes, or hospitals get very little direct sun exposure. Dark skinned persons require 10 to 15 times the same sun exposure to produce equivalent amounts of vitamin D than in light skinned persons. Melanin absorbs UV radiation and competes for UVB photons that are needed for vitamin D production. [8] Air pollution and clothing that covers the entire body, as required in some cultures, also reduces UVB exposure. Additionally, obesity impacts the amount of circulating vitamin D that is produced in the skin as subcutaneous fat sequesters the synthesized vitamin D in its cells making it unavailable for conversion to $1,25(OH)_2$ D [2].

Figure 1. Skin—Principal Source of Vitamin D Production.

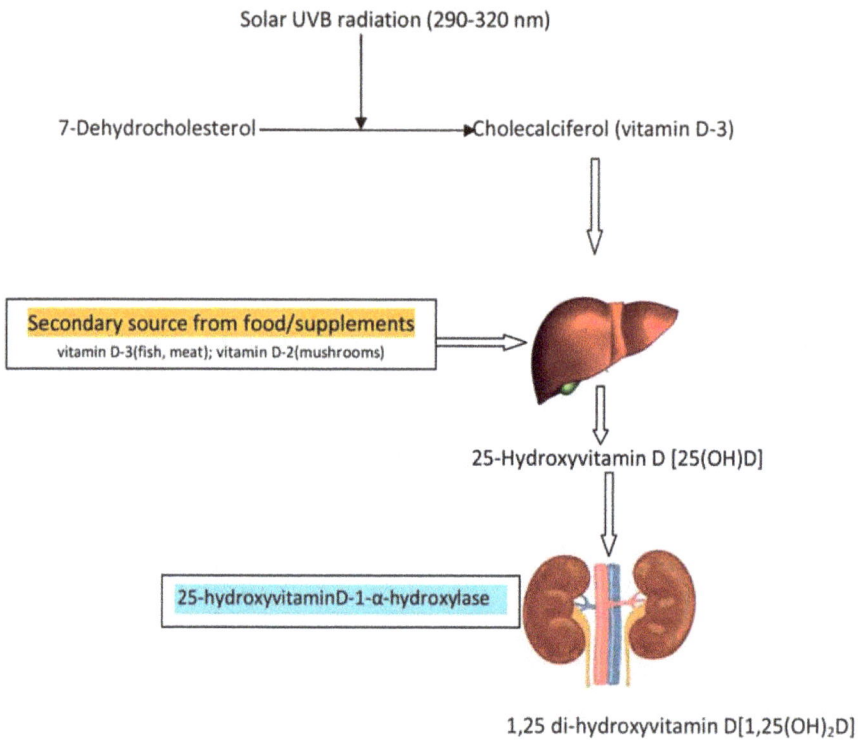

Solar UVB radiation (290-320 nm)

7-Dehydrocholesterol ⟶ Cholecalciferol (vitamin D-3)

Secondary source from food/supplements
vitamin D-3(fish, meat); vitamin D-2(mushrooms)

25-Hydroxyvitamin D [25(OH)D]

25-hydroxyvitaminD-1-α-hydroxylase

1,25 di-hydroxyvitamin D[$1,25(OH)_2$D]

Conversion of 25(OH)D to $1,25(OH)_2$D in the kidney is tightly regulated by PTH, calcium, and phosphorus levels

Certain medications and medical conditions can also affect the amount of circulating vitamin D. Drugs that are dependent on the cytochrome P-450 system for metabolism, such as phenobarbital, valproic acid, and ketoconazole, compete with Vitamin D for this pathway. Drug-vitamin studies have shown a decrease in vitamin D levels with use of these medications. Malabsorption disorders, such as cystic fibrosis or Crohn's disease, liver disease, and kidney disease, also affect vitamin D levels and utilization [4].

2.2. Measurement of Vitamin D Levels

Deciding which vitamin D level to measure depends on what needs to be assessed clinically. 25(OH)D, though metabolically inactive, is the major circulating from of vitamin D. It is generally the best indicator of overall vitamin D status and is used to correlate vitamin D stores with clinical disease. The circulating half-life is 2 to 3 weeks (Table 1). 1,25(OH)$_2$D, the metabolically active form, is closely regulated by 25(OH)D, PTH, calcium and phosphorus, and is measured to assess calcium metabolic disorders related to the renal production of 1,25(OH)$_2$D. Its circulating half-life is 4 to 6 hours.

Low 25 (OH)D levels lead to decreased intestinal absorption of calcium causing a transient decrease of ionized calcium. This signals an increase of PTH to mobilize calcium from bones, increase tubular reabsorption of calcium from the kidneys, and increase production of 1,25(OH)$_2$D by the kidneys. This increased production of 1,25(OH)D$_2$D may not always need to occur, therefore low 25(OH)D may be associated with normal or elevated 1,25(OH)$_2$D levels [4].

Table 1. Current accepted definitions of various Vitamin D levels include: [9].

>150 ng/mL	**Toxicity**
100 ng/mL	Maximum upper limit
40–70 ng/mL	Ideal range
>30 ng/mL	Sufficient
21–29 ng/mL	Insufficient
<20 ng/mL	Deficient

Vitamin D intoxication is defined as a 25(OH)D level >150 ng/mL associated with hypercalcemia, hypercalciuria, and hyperphosphatemia. Sunlight destroys excess vitamin D that is produced in the body so it is not possible to get vitamin D intoxication from sun exposure alone. Studies on outdoor workers during summer months found naturally produced vitamin D levels averaged around 50 ng/mL. Lifeguards at the beach had reported levels of 100 to 125 ng/mL without evidence of toxicity [10]. Toxicity could potentially occur with supplementation with vitamin D of greater than 10,000 IU daily over a prolonged period of time.

Vitamin D intoxication did occur in children who received an erroneously manufactured dietary supplement of fish oil with added vitamin D. These children presented with symptoms of hypercalcemia—weakness, constipation, loss of appetite, nausea, vomiting—and found to have serum calcium levels of 13.4 to 18.8 mg/dL. They also had measured levels of 25(OH)D of 340 to 962 ng/mL. When supplement intake was discovered and the product tested, the vitamin D was 4,000 times its stated amount. Estimated intakes of vitamin D for these children were between 266,000 to 800,000 IU per day. With discontinuation of the dietary supplement and with treatment, calcium levels normalized within 3 days and 25(OH)D levels normalized within 2–3 months [11].

On the other hand, insufficient and deficient levels, <30 ng/mL and <20 ng/mL respectfully, are commonly found in the general population. A recent National Health and Nutrition Examination Survey (NHANES) estimated that 10.3% of US children aged 6–18 years (population estimate 5.5 million) have 25(OH)D levels <16 ng/mL. Generally, vitamin D levels were lowest in

African-American children averaging 20 ng/mL and Hispanics at 24 ng/mL. Most of these children showed some evidence of bone demineralization on standard radiographs [12,13]. It is unclear if this was related specifically to skin pigment, diet, or lifestyle or combination thereof.

Only 10% to 15% of dietary calcium and 60% of dietary phosphorus is absorbed from the intestinal tract in low vitamin D states. When 25(OH)D levels fall below 40 ng/mL, PTH is activated due to the decrease in calcium absorption from the intestines. PTH activates osteoblasts that stimulate the formation of osteoclasts which dissolve the calcium: phosphorus collagen matrix in bone. If not remedied, this can lead to osteopenia and rickets. The incidence of rickets in the industrialized world has increased over the past two decades as documented in the US, Canada, and Australia [14–16]. Rickets is most prevalent in darker pigmented races (immigrant refugees), in those living at higher latitudes, and in breast or formula fed babies who do not receive adequate vitamin D supplementation.

Vitamin D experts advocate targeting 25(OH)D levels of 40 to 70 ng/mL to achieve the optimal skeletal function without toxicity [3,9]. Maintaining 25(OH)D levels above 40 ng/mL keeps PTH suppressed and allows for most favorable absorption of calcium from the intestines. Beyond the skeletal benefits, studies are now showing a correlation of improved health outcomes with higher levels of vitamin D. Advocating for vitamin D levels to reach the optimal levels noted above has been controversial and there have been conflicting recommendations since the release of the 2010 IOM report on vitamin D supplementation. This report stated that the recommended daily allowance (RDA) of 600 IU is the upper limit that should be given to any child or adult regardless of measured blood levels [17]. Based on pooled published studies, however, primarily in adults, the disease incidence prevention from higher 25(OH)D levels was significant. This could have important implications in preventative health care for children Figure 2 [18].

Figure 2. Disease Incidence Prevention by serum 25(OH)D levels. [18] (Used with permission).

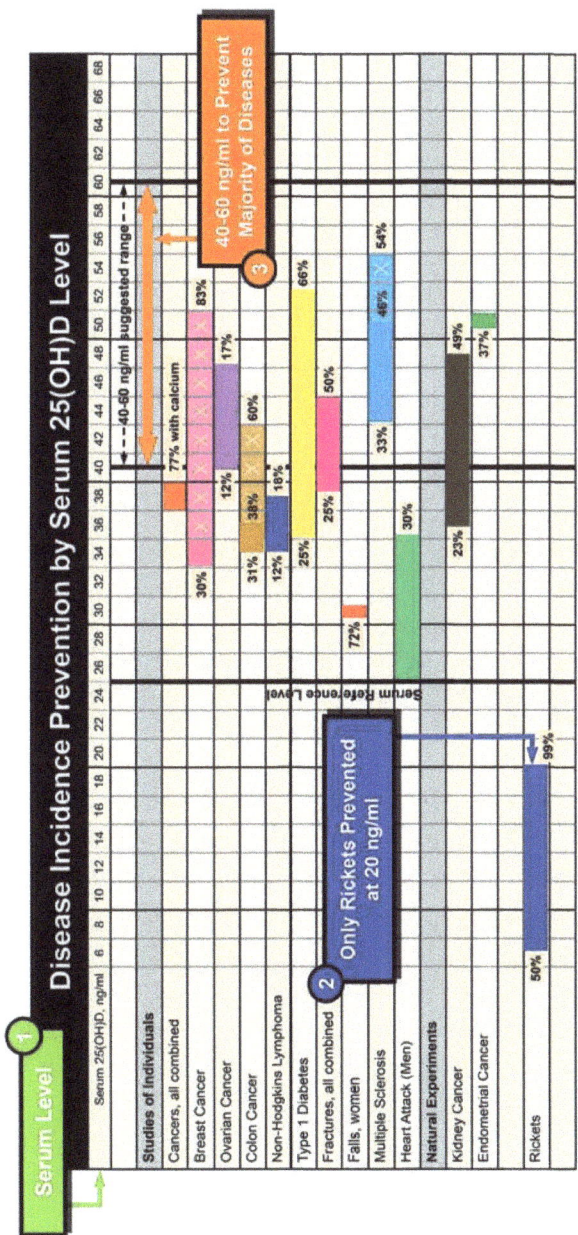

Chart prepared by: Garland CF, Baggerly CA

Legend:
All percentages reference a common baseline of 25 ng/ml as shown on the chart.
%'s reflect the disease prevention % at the beginning and ending of available data. Example: Breast cancer incidence is reduced by 30% when the serum level is 34 ng/ml vs the baseline of 25 ng/ml. There is an 83% reduction in incidence when the serum level is 50 ng/ml vs the baseline of 25 ng/ml.
The x's in the bars indicate 'reasonable extrapolations from the data but are beyond existing data.

References:
All Cancers: Lappe JM, et al. Am J Clin Nutr 2007;85:1586-91. Breast: Garland CF, Gorham ED, Mohr SB, Grant WB, Garland FC. Breast cancer risk according to serum 25-Hydroxyvitamin D: Meta-analysis of Dose-Response (abstract). American Association for Cancer Research Annual Meeting, 2008. Reference serum 25(OH)D was 5 ng/ml. Garland, CF, et al. Amer Assoc Cancer Research Annual Mtg, April 2008. Colon: Gorham ED, et al. Am J Prev Med. 2007:32:210-6. Diabetes: Hyppönen E, et al. Lancet 2001;358:1500-3. Endometrium: Mohr SB, et al. Prev Med. 2007;45:323-4. Falls: Broe KE, et al. J Am Geriatr Soc. 2007;55:234-9. Fractures: Bischoff-Ferrari HA, et al. JAMA. 2005;293:2257-64. Heart Attack: Giovannucci et al. Arch Intern Med/Vol 168 (No 11) June 9, 2008. Multiple Sclerosis: Munger KL, et al. JAMA. 2006;296:2832-8. Non-Hodgkin's Lymphoma: Purdue MP. et al. Cancer Causes Control. 2007:18:989-99. Ovary: Tworoger SS, et al. Cancer Epidemiol Biomarkers Prev. 2007:16:783-8. Renal: Mohr SB, et al. Int J Cancer. 2006;119:2705-9. Rickets: Arnaud SB, et al. Pediatrics 1976 Feb;57(2):221-5.

2.3. Extraskeletal Effects of Vitamin D

Vitamin D is known to have direct effects on innate immunity. Vitamin D receptors (VDR) are present in lymphocytes, monocytes and macrophages. In TB infections, for example, immune cells up-regulate their own expression of VDR and 1-α-hydroxylase increasing the local production of 1,25(OH)$_2$D. This activates the transcription of antimicrobial peptides, cathelicidins and defensins [6]. When serum 25(OH)D levels fall below 20 ng/mL, monocytes and macrophages cannot initiate the innate immune response [19]. This activation of antimicrobial peptides also occurs in the skin and epithelial cells throughout the body. Localized injury or insult of the mucocutaneous barrier by viruses or bacteria activates 1-α-hydroxylase in tissues thereby increasing the local production of 1,25(OH)$_2$D. This augments the expression of tissue cathelicidins and defensins thereby producing antimicrombial effects at the site of insult. The fact that the incidence of upper respiratory illnesses and influenza is higher after the winter solstice, in higher latitudes, in children with rickets, and in the institutionalized again seems to support the theory that the lack of vitamin D increases susceptibility to illness. In a study on vitamin D and osteoporosis in adults, those participants with low vitamin D levels were 40% more likely to report a recent URI compared to those whose 25(OH)D levels were > 30 ng/mL [20].

Prospective trials have been done studying the effects of vitamin D on the incidence of microbial illness in children. One study found an inverse association between cord-blood levels of 25 (OH)D and the risk of developing infections in infants. Newborns with 25(OH)D levels of <10 ng/mL were more likely to develop upper respiratory infections or otitis media by 3 months of age and wheezing at 15 months compared to those who had higher levels [21]. Cord blood vitamin D deficiency in otherwise healthy neonates was also associated with an increased risk of developing respiratory syncytial virus (RSV) during infancy. Neonates born with 25(OH)D concentrations <20 ng/mL had a six fold increased risk of developing a lower respiratory tract infection with RSV in the first year of life compared with those with 25(OH)D concentrations ≥30 ng/mL [22]. A randomized controlled trial compared the use of 1200 IU of vitamin D to placebo in 334 Japanese children during the months of December through March on the incidence of influenza A. The outcomes showed the study group was 58% less likely to get influenza A compared to the placebo group. Additionally, of the children who also had asthma, only 2 in the study group *vs.* 12 in the placebo group contracted influenza A [23].

Vitamin D also plays a role in adaptive immunity with nuclear VDR and vitamin D-activating enzymes present in both T and B cells. In the presence of vitamin D, T cells inhibit the secretion of pro-inflammatory Th-1 cytokines (IL-2, interferon γ, TNF-α) and promotes the production of the more anti-inflammatory Th-2 cytokines (IL-3, 4, 5, 10). Vitamin D also controls B-cell activation and proliferation thus reducing the production of auto-reactive antibodies [24]. This is important as epidemiological studies have shown an association between vitamin D deficiency and the increased incidence of autoimmune diseases. Many of these diseases, such as multiple sclerosis (MS), rheumatoid arthritis (RA), Crohn's disease, and Type 1 diabetes mellitus (DM), are more prevalent in populations residing in higher latitudes. Women living at 35° N latitude for the first 10 years of life had an almost 100% increased risk of developing MS [25]. Women at this same latitude who took >400 IU of Vitamin D daily had a 42% decreased risk of developing MS [26]. Ten thousand three hundred sixty-six children in Finland received 2,000 IU of Vitamin D daily for the first year of life and then followed for the next 31 years. These children had a 78% reduced risk of developing Type 1 DM compared to those who did not receive this supplementation [27].

It is suggested that both MS and Type 1 DM may be caused by viral infections early in life. These infections trigger the destruction of myelin (in MS) and islet cells (in DM) from the action of excess pro-inflammatory cytokines and autoantibodies found in low vitamin D states. Increasing vitamin D intake during pregnancy reduced the development of islet cell auto-antibodies in offspring, thus supporting aspects of this theory [28].

The benefit of adequate vitamin D has also been demonstrated in children with asthma, eczema, and allergies. One thousand ninety-four mother-child pairs were evaluated for vitamin D levels and the incidence of childhood wheezing. Mothers with the highest intake of vitamin D were 61% less likely to have a child with recurrent wheeze, and for each 100 IU increase of intake, the risk fell by 19% [29].

A RCT compared the use of budesonide alone to budesonide plus daily supplementation with vitamin D 500 IU in children newly diagnosed with asthma. At six months, both groups had significant improvements in lung function as measured by FEV-1 and the Asthma Therapy Assessment Questionnaire (ATAQ). There were significantly fewer asthma exacerbations, however, in the vitamin D group compared to the budesonide only group. It was noted that each exacerbation was precede by an acute respiratory infection thereby it was surmised that vitamin D intake reduced the incidence of acute URI that triggered asthma exacerbations [30].

Children with eczema who took vitamin D 4000 IU daily for 21 days had significant increases in cathelecidin levels and reduced colonization of skin pathogens [31]. Low vitamin D levels correlated with sensitivity to 11 of 17 allergens tested via IgE RAST for food and environmental triggers. Children with 25(OH)D levels <15 ng/mL were more likely to have peanut, ragweed and oak allergy [32].

2.4. Vitamin D and Cancer

Practically all tissues express 1-α-hydroxylase that allows for local production of 1,25(OH)$_2$D. This, in turn controls the local expression of genes that regulate cell proliferation and differentiation. It is known that activated vitamin D blocks cells at the G-1 phase, modulates production of several pro-oncogenes, and promotes apoptosis in some forms of cancer. Activated vitamin D also decreases angiogensis which reduces the risk of dissemination [33].

The majority of studies evaluating the association of vitamin D levels to cancer found a protective relationship between sufficient vitamin D status and lower risk of cancer [34]. People living at higher latitudes show an increase risk for developing Hodgkin's lymphoma, pancreatic, breast, colon, and ovarian cancers. When compared to patients with these same diseases living at lower latitudes, those at higher latitudes were more likely to die, even when controlled for lifestyle. These statistics were associated with 25(OH)D levels <20 ng/mL [35]. In another epidemiological study, children and young adults exposed to the most sunlight had a 40% reduced risk of developing non-Hodgkin's lymphoma [36].

Overall there is a strong inverse correlation for solar UVB irradiance and the incidence of various cancers—bladder, breast, cervical, colon, endometrial, esophageal, gastric, lung, ovarian, pancreatic, rectal, renal, vulvar, and Hodgkin's and non-Hodgkin's lymphoma. This same effect was not found with vitamin D oral supplementation [37].

The campaign for use of sun-screens and for sun avoidance was initiated to reduce the incidence of skin cancers. Though this has decreased some forms of non-melanoma cancer, the actual rate of melanoma has increased [38]. The working theory to explain this phenomenon suggests that sunscreens primarily block UVB rays to prevent sunburn, but do not fully block UVA or UVC rays that penetrate the deeper layers of skin causing DNA damage. With the reduced risk of sun burn, individuals often have prolonged sun exposures not realizing that deeper damage is occurring.

2.5. Vitamin D and Pain

Vitamin D increases muscle protein synthesis, possibly by activating second messengers and phosphorylation [39]. In mouse models, skeletal muscle hypersensitivity with increased numbers of nociceptor axions were documented in mice with vitamin D deficient states but not in those with vitamin D sufficient states [40]. Vitamin D deficiency has been associated with muscle pain and proximal muscle weakness with reports of heaviness in the legs, rapid fatigue, and problems with climbing stairs or mobility. Vitamin D deficiency is also frequently documented in patients diagnosed with fibromyalgia and non-specific musculoskeletal pain [41]. In pediatrics, vitamin D deficiency may present as atypical muscular pain and is found more typically in those who are Caucasian, have a history of being breastfed, are protected from the sun, and are obese [42].

In a recent clinical study of individuals with chronic pain, 71% of enrolled subjects were vitamin D deficient (<20 ng/mL) and 21% were vitamin D insufficient (20–30 ng/mL). Only 8% of these subjects had levels > 30 ng/mL. Lower vitamin D levels were significantly associated with higher pain sensitivity scores [43]. In another study, resolution of pain occurred when subjects with chronic pain were adequately supplemented with vitamin D-3 to reach 25-hydroxy Vitamin D levels of >30 ng/mL [44].

Very low vitamin D levels have been found in a survey of children with migraine as well [45]. Vitamin D deficiency is associated with higher levels of pro-inflammatory and pro-coagulatory biomarkers—some of the same biomarkers known to be elevated in adult and pediatric patients with migraine. These biomarkers are indicative of endothelial activation and vascular reactivity caused by inflammation and oxidative stress [46,47]. Vitamin D, because of its immune modulation, nerve stabilizing, and antithrombotic effects may decrease the incidence of migraine. Thus far no randomized, placebo controlled studies have been conducted in adults or children using vitamin D to prevent or treat migraine, however several case reports suggest that vitamin D may be effective in reducing migraine pain in adults. There was demonstrated reduction of headache pain when patients were supplemented with vitamin D (1000–1500 IU) and calcium (1000–1500 mg). Though the role of calcium in suppressing pain could not be ruled out, vitamin D seemingly was more vital for headache relief. Serum calcium levels normalized within the first week of therapy, but headache pain only abated once there was normalization of the 25(OH)D levels which occurred at 4 to 6 weeks of treatment [48].

2.6. Vitamin D and Mental Health

Vitamin D is emerging as a steroid derivative with neuroactive properties that have direct effects on brain development. There is a wide distribution of VDR and 1-α-hydroxylase throughout the brain allowing for local production of activated vitamin D. 1,25(OH)$_2$D regulates nerve growth factor and glial cell line-derived neurotropic factor which orchestrates the cellular architecture of the brain. Activated vitamin D also has neuroprotective effects via neuromodulation, anti-inflammatory, anti-ischemic, and anti-oxidant properties [6].

Having adequate vitamin D levels in-utero and early stages of life ensures normal receptor transcriptional activity vital for brain development and mental functioning [49]. Vitamin D affects the proteins directly involved in learning, memory, motor control, and social behavior [50], and is closely associated with executive functioning such as goal-directed behavior, attention, and adaptability to change [51].

Vitamin D deficiency and insufficiency are found frequently in adolescents with severe mental illness. Vitamin D deficiency has been linked to an increased risk of developing schizophrenia. In one study of adolescents admitted to an acute mental health facility, those who were vitamin D deficient were 3½ times more likely to have psychotic features when compared to vitamin D sufficient patients [52]. In another review of psychiatric patients, those with the lowest levels of vitamin D (<20 ng/mL) were more likely to be male, of Middle East, South-East Asian, or African ethnicity, and had diagnoses of autism and schizophrenia. When supplemented with 1000 to 4000 IU of vitamin D, many had clinical improvement [53].

Vitamin D deficiency has also been associated with depression and seasonal effective disorder. Vitamin D deficiency decreases the expression of the enzyme catechol-O-methyl transferase (COMT), required for dopamine and serotonin metabolism. This has been associated with negative CNS effects in animal studies [50]. In human studies, resolution of depression occurred when depressed adolescents were adequately supplemented with vitamin D-3 to reach 25(OH)D levels of >30 ng/mL [54].

There has been an undeniable increase in the incidence of autism since the 1980s that is not explained by changes in diagnostic criteria or changes in reporting. The incidence of autism in 1980 was approximately 1:200 but now stands at 1:68 in the US [55]. Studies in Asia, Europe, and North America have identified individuals with autism with an average prevalence of about 1%. A study in South Korea reported a prevalence of 2.6% [56]. Current research suggests that autism may have an underlying genetic susceptibility with biochemical abnormalities. This susceptible state is impacted by environmental influences which trigger the development of autism through mitochondrial dysfunction, immune dysregulation, inflammation, oxidative stress, methylation problems, and toxicity [57].

The lack of adequate vitamin D, in theory, may play a role in the development of autism (Table 2). What is currently known:

Also known is the strong correlation between latitude and the incidence of autism, increased number of children with autism born during the winter months, more autistic children are born to multiparous women, higher prevalence of autism in geographic areas with highest cloud cover and

46

precipitation, and greater incidence in urban *vs.* rural populations (possibly from air pollution, tall buildings, indoor living) [68–71]. The vitamin D theory does not diminish the genetic or other environmental contributions; rather it may allow the genetic tendency of autism to express itself in a state of vitamin D deficiency.

Table 2. Commonalities between Autism and Vitamin D deficiency.

Autism	Vitamin D
Serotonin, which promotes social behavior and facilitates accurate assessment of emotional social cues, is reduced in autistic brains. Low Vitamin D levels are also commonly found in autism.	1,25(OH)$_2$D activates the transcription of tryptophan hydroxylase-2, an enzyme that converts tryptophan to serotonin in the brain [58].
Increased levels of inflammatory cytokines are found in autism-- IL-1β, IL-6, IL-8, *etc* [59]	Inflammatory cytokines (IL-6, IL-10, CRP, *etc*) are elevated in Vitamin D deficiency [60].
Low glutathione levels found in autism—difficulty excreting heavy metals [61].	Vitamin D increases glutathione in the brain—suggesting a role for the hormone in brain detoxification pathways [62].
Depakote has been associated with autism in children of mothers taking this during pregnancy [63].	Depakote lowers Vitamin D levels [64].
Seizures are common in children with autism [65].	Normalization of serum vitamin 25(OH)D level has an anticonvulsant effect [66].
Autism occurs more frequently in male > females.	Estrogen protects the developing female brain from Vitamin D deficiency (oxidative stress). Testosterone does not [67].

2.7. Vitamin D in Pregnancy and Effects on Fetus and Newborn

Vitamin D deficiency and insufficiency occur in 27% to 91% of all pregnant women depending on the country of residence [7]. A meta-analysis of studies assessing vitamin D in pregnancy showed an inverse association of low vitamin D levels and the risk of pre-eclampsia, gestational diabetes, pre-term births, and small for gestational age babies [72]. Low maternal vitamin D predisposes the fetus/newborn to low vitamin D stores as well leading to rickets, wheezing, and upper respiratory tract infections and mental health issues as noted before. Vitamin D deficiency in pregnancy has also been associated with the increased development of IgE-specific allergens and eczema in offspring [73,74]. An Australian study found maternal vitamin D insufficiency during pregnancy was associated with language impairment in their offspring [75]. Yet another study found inadequate vitamin D during pregnancy effected tooth calcification in the newborn. Women who had the lowest 25 (OH)D levels had children with a greater incidence of tooth enamel hypoplasia and early childhood caries by age 1 year [76].

Exclusive breastfeeding without adequate sun exposure or vitamin D supplementation contributes to ongoing vitamin D deficiency in newborns as unsupplemented breast milk only contains 20 to 80 IU/L of vitamin D. (By comparison, infant formula is required to be fortified with 40 to 100 IU of vitamin D per 100 kcal to give approximately 270 to 677 IU/L.) Research revealed that lactating women often need 25 (OH)D levels of 40 to 50 ng/mL to provide sufficient vitamin D in breast milk for nursing infants [77]. Daily doses of 4000 to 5000 IU daily of cholecalciferol (Vitamin D-3) were required to achieve optimal 25(OH)D serum levels in lactating women and did not cause toxicity [78,79]. This dose is much higher than the recommended daily allowance of 600 IU suggested by the IOM for adults and lactating women and also significantly higher than the amount of vitamin D found in standard pre-natal or multivitamins which typically provide 400 to 600 IU per dose.

2.8. Recommended Supplementation

Being aware of the risk factors associated with the development of vitamin D deficiency will help guide clinicians to both assess for and intervene with supplementation as needed.

- Infants who are exclusively breast fed or ingest less than 1000 mL of infant formula a day
- Children living north or south of the 33° latitudes or in urban/polluted environments
- Those that are obese, deeply pigmented or, for cultural reasons, cover their skin with clothing
- Those with disorders of digestion or who are on medications that prevents absorption of vitamin D
- Children who are institutionalized, hospitalized, or attend schools that limit outside play

One can choose to measure 25(OH)D levels to document vitamin D deficiency, but with the widespread findings of insufficiency and deficiency in most cultures, it is relatively safe to start vitamin D supplementation without this information.

Supplementing with natural sunlight 15 to 30 min a day during the hours of 10 AM to 3 PM is optimal for prevention and treatment of vitamin D deficiency; however, this may not be available to all those at risk. Vitamin D-3 (cholecalciferol) or vitamin D-2 (ergocalciferol) are both available for oral supplementation and both are transformed in the liver and kidneys to the active $1,25(OH)_2D$. Research has found, however, that Vitamin D3 is approximately 87 percent more potent in raising and maintaining vitamin D concentrations and produces a 2- to 3-fold greater storage of vitamin D than does vitamin D2 [80].

Supplementing 400 IU daily of Vitamin D3, as recommended by the American Academy of Pediatrics (AAP) and the IOM, or up to 800 IU as recommended by the Canadian Pediatric Society may provide sufficient vitamin D to prevent rickets, but higher doses may be needed to achieve other health benefits [81]. For every 100 IU intake of vitamin D3, serum levels increase by 1 ng/mL when given over 3 to 4 months [82]. For a child who is deficient, a standard dose of 400 IU will not correct this problem. A study of breast fed infants found that only a dose of 1600 IU/day (and not 400, 800, or 1200 IU) could raise 25(OH)D to a level >28 ng/mL after 3 months [83]. It is recommended by experts in the field of vitamin D research that healthy children receive approximately 1000 IU per 11 Kg of body weight each day to achieve optimal 25(OH)D levels year round [84]. Having a baseline 25(OH)D level can help guide initial dosing with a follow- up level in 2 to 3 months to monitor efficacy.

2.9. Potential Economic Impact

Given the high incidence of vitamin D insufficiency/deficiency, convincing evidence for benefit, and the strong evidence of safety, vitamin D supplementation should be utilized more now than ever. Interest groups and researchers have been advocating for education on vitamin D deficiency and for wide-spread vitamin D supplementation to reduce the burden of disease. Despite these efforts, vitamin D deficiency and its sequellae persist [85].

Grant *et al.* assessed the economic burden and premature death related to vitamin D deficiency in North America and estimated what would change if 25(OH)D levels were optimized in all individuals. They used data from studies that demonstrated significant vitamin D effects on disease incidence or mortality rates. From these studies, they estimated that all-cancer incidence rates would decrease approximately 25%, influenza and pneumonia rates would decrease approximately 30%, septicemia would decrease 25%, multiple sclerosis by 40%, and negative pregnancy outcomes (including asthma, infections, bone disorders, heart failure, and autism in the offspring) would be reduced by 10% [86]. In assessing the overall cost savings in Canada alone, they estimated the death rate would fall by 16% and that the total economic burden would decrease by 6.9% or approximately $14.4 billion per year.

Estimated annual costs of various diseases influenced by vitamin D in the United States are listed below (Table 3).

Table 3. Estimated annual costs of common disorders that potentially could be attenuated by adequate Vitamin D levels.

Disease	Direct (in US Dollars)	Indirect (in US Dollars)	Total Annual Expense (US)
Influenza	10.4 billion	16.3 billion	26.7 billion [87]
Asthma	50.1 billion	5.9 billion	56 billion [88]
Upper respiratory infections	17 billion	23.5 billion	40 billion [89]
Autism	—	—	126 billion [90]
Cancer	86.6 billion	130 billion	216.6 billion [91]

If one used the same data from Grant's study, the saving of life and money could be even greater in the United States which has almost 10 times the population of Canada. With a current population near 320 million, supplementing each person in the US with 3000 IU per day of vitamin D3 to achieve optimal 25(OH)D levels would cost approximately $3 billion per year (based on current retail costs found on the Internet of approximately $10 per year). This relatively low cost intervention could potentially save $84 billion dollars in total health care costs just for these diseases alone.

3. Conclusions

Beyond the skeletal effects it pro-offers, there is more evidence now supporting the beneficial benefits vitamin D has on immune health, mental health, and overall life expectancy. For the sake of public health, instituting a proactive program, much like the current immunization programs, using vitamin D supplementation could have dramatic impact on overall health worldwide by reducing the physical, emotional, and economic burden of disease.

Acknowledgments

I would like to thank Thomas M. Fine for reviewing this manuscript and for providing editorial comments.

Author Contributions

J.W. contributed to the entire content of this manuscript.

Conflicts of Interest

The author declares no conflict of interest.

References

1. Pub Med. Available online: http://www.ncbi.nlm.nih.gov (accessed on 1 September 2014).
2. Holick, M.F. Vitamin D deficiency. *N. Engl. J. Med.* **2007**, *357*, 266–281.
3. Cannell, J.J.; Hollis, B.W. Use of vitamin D in clinical practice. *Altern. Med. Rev.* **2008**, *13*, 6–20.
4. Holick, M.F. The Vitamin D deficiency pandemic and consequences for non-skeletal health: Mechanism of action. *Mol. Aspect Med.* **2008**, *29*, 362–368.
5. Lips, P. Vitamin D physiology. *Prog. Biophys. Mol. Biol.* **2006**, *92*, 4–8.
6. Bouvard, B.; Annweiler, C.; Sallé, A.; Beauchet, O.; Chappard, D.; Audran, M.; Legrand, E. Extraskeletal effects of vitamin D: Facts, uncertainties, and controversies. *Joint Bone Spine* **2011**, *78*, 10–16.
7. Hossein-nezhad, A.; Holick, M.F. Vitamin D for health: A global perspective. *Mayo Clin. Proc.* **2013**, *88*, 720–755.
8. Holick, M.F. Environmental factors that influence the cutaneous production of vitamin D. *Am. J. Clin. Nutr.* **1995**, *61*, 638S–645S.
9. Vasquez, A.; Manso, G.; Cannell, J. The clinical importance of vitamin D (cholecalciferol): A paradigm shift with implications for all healthcare providers. *Altern. Ther. Health Med.* **2004**, *10*, 28–36.
10. Barger-Lux, M.J.; Heaney, R.P. Effects of above average summer sun exposure on serum 25-hydroxyvitamin D and calcium absorption. *J. Clin. Endocrinol. Metab.* **2002**, *87*, 4952–4956.
11. Kara, C.; Gunindi, F.; Ustyol, A.; Aydin, M. Vitamin D intoxication due to an erroneously manufactured dietary supplement in seven children. *Pediatrics* **2014**, *133*, e240–e244.
12. Kumar, J.; Muntner, P.; Kaskel, F.J.; Hailpern, S.M.; Melamed, M.L. Prevalence and associations of 25-hydroxyvitamin D deficiency in US children: NHANES 2001–2004. *Pediatrics* **2009**, *124*, e362–e370.
13. Karalius, V.P.; Zinn, D.; Wu, J.; *et al.* Prevalence of risk of deficiency and inadequacy of 25-hydroxyvitamin D in US children: NHANES 2003–2006. *J. Pediatr. Endocrinol. Metab.* **2014**, *27*, 461–466.

14. Thacher, T.D.; Fischer, P.R.; Tebben, P.J.; Singh, R.J.; Cha, S.S.; Maxson, J.A.; Yawn, B.P. Increasing incidence of nutritional rickets: A population-based study in Olmsted County, Minnesota. *Mayo Clin. Proc.* **2013**, *88*, 176–183.
15. Ward, L.E.; Gaboury, I.; Ladhani, M.; Zlotkin, S. Vitamin D-deficiency rickets among children in Canada. *CMAJ* **2007**, *177*, 161–166.
16. Munns, C.F.; Simm, P.J.; Rodda, C.P.; Garnett, S.P.; Zacharin, M.R.; Ward, L.M.; Geddes, J.; Cherian, S.; Zurynski, Y.; Cowell, C.T.; *et al.* Incidence of vitamin D deficiency rickets among Australian children: An Australian Paediatric Surveillance Unit study. *Med. J. Aust.* **2012**, *196*, 466–468.
17. Ross, A.C.; Abrams, S.A.; Aloia, J.F.; Brannon, P.M.; Clinton, S.K.; Durazo-Arvizu, R.A.; Gallagher, J.C.; Gallo, R.L.; Jones, G.; Kovacs, C.S.; *et al.* Dietary Reference Intakes for Calcium and Vitamin D. National Academy of Sciences, Institute of Medicine: Washington, DC, USA. Available online: http://www.iom.edu/Reports/2010/Dietary-Reference-Intakes-for-Calcium-and-Vitamin-D.aspx (accessed on 1 September, 2014).
18. GrassrootsHealth. Available online: http://www.grassrootshealth.net (accessed on 1 September 2014).
19. Liu, P.T.; Stenger, S.; Li, H.; Wenzel, L.; Tan, B.H.; Krutzik, S.R.; Ochoa, M.T.; Schauber, J.; Wu, K.; Meinken, C.; *et al.* Toll-like receptor triggering of a vitamin D-mediated human antimicrobial response. *Science* **2006**, *311*, 1770–1773.
20. Ginde, A.A.; Mansbach, J.M.; Camargo, C. Association between serum 25-hydroxyvitamin D level and upper respiratory tract infection in the Third National Health and Nutrition Examination Survey. *Arch. Intern. Med.* **2009**, *69*, 384–390.
21. Camargo, C.A.; Ingham, T.; Wickens, K.; Thadhani, R.; Silvers, K.M.; Epton, M.J.; Town, G.I.; Pattemore, P.K.; Espinola, J.A.; Crane, J.; *et al.* Cord-blood 25-hydroxyvitamin D levels and risk of respiratory infection, wheezing, and asthma. *Pediatrics* **2011**, *127*, e180–e187.
22. Belderbos, M.E.; Houben, M.L.; Wilbrink, B.; Lentjes, E.; Bloemen, E.M.; Kimpen, J.L.; Rovers, M.; Bont, L. Cord blood vitamin D deficiency is associated with respiratory syncytial virus bronchiolitis. *Pediatrics* **2011**, *127*, e1513–e1520.
23. Urashima, M.; Segawa, T.; Okazaki, M.; Kurihara, M.; Wada, Y.; Ida, H. Randomized trial of vitamin D supplementation to prevent seasonal influenza A in schoolchildren. *Am. J. Clin. Nutr.* **2010**, *91*, 1255–1260.
24. Prietl, B.; Treiber, G.; Pieber, T.R.; Amrein, K. Vitamin D and immune function. *Nutrients* **2013**, *5*, 2502–2521.
25. Ponsonby, A.L.; McMichael, A.; van der Mei, I. Ultraviolet radiation and autoimmune disease: Insights from epidemiological research. *Toxicology* **2002**, *181–182*, 71–78.
26. Munger, K.L.; Zhang, S.M.; O'Reilly, E.; Hernán, M.A.; Olek, M.J.; Willett, W.C.; Ascherio, A. Vitamin D intake and incidence of multiple sclerosis. *Neurology* **2004**, *62*, 60–65.
27. Hyppönen, E.; Läärä, E.; Reunanen, A.; Järvelin, M.R.; Virtanen, S.M. Intake of vitamin D and risk of type 1 diabetes: A birth-cohort study. *Lancet* **2001**, *358*, 1500–1503.
28. Chiu, K.C.; Chu, A.; Go, V.L.; Saad, M.F. Hypovitaminosis D is associated with insulin resistance and beta cell dysfunction. *Am. J. Clin. Nutr.* **2004**, *79*, 820–825.

29. Camargo, C.A.; Rifas-Shiman, S.L.; Litonjua, A.A. Maternal intake of vitamin D during pregnancy and risk of recurrent wheeze in children at 3 y of age. *Am. J. Clin. Nutr.* **2007**, *85*, 788–795.

30. Majak, P.; Olszowiec-Chlebna, M.; Smejda, K.; Stelmach, I. Vitamin D supplementation in children may prevent asthma exacerbation triggered by acute respiratory infection. *J. Allergy Clin. Immunol.* **2011**, *127*, 1294–1296.

31. Hata, T.R.; Kotol, P.; Jackson, M.; Nguyen, M.; Paik, A.; Udall, D.; Kanada, K.; Yamasaki, K.; Alexandrescu, D.; Gallo, R.L. Administration of oral vitamin D induces cathelicidin production in atopic individuals. *J. Allergy Clin. Immunol.* **2008**, *122*, 829–831.

32. Sharief, S.; Jariwala, S.; Kumar, J.; Muntner, P.; Melamed, M.L. Vitamin D levels and food and environmental allergies in the United States: Results from the National Health and Nutrition Examination Survey 2005–2006. *J. Allergy Clin. Immunol.* **2011**, *27*, 1195–1202.

33. Ooi, L.L.; Zhou, H.; Kalak, R.; Zheng, Y.; Conigrave, A.D.; Seibel, M.J.; Dunstan, C.R. Vitamin D deficiency promotes human breast cancer growth in a murine model of bone metastasis. *Cancer Res.* **2010**, *70*, 1835–1844.

34. Garland, C.F.; Garland, F.C.; Gorham, E.D.; Lipkin, M.; Newmark, H.; Mohr, S.B.; Holick, M.F. The role of vitamin D in cancer prevention. *Am. J. Public Health* **2006**, *96*, 252–261.

35. Grant, W.B. An estimate of premature cancer mortality in the U.S. due to inadequate doses of solar ultraviolet-B radiation. *Cancer* **2002**, *94*, 1867–1875.

36. Smedby, K.E.; Hjalgrim, H.; Melbye, M.; Torrång, A.; Rostgaard, K.; Munksgaard, L.; Adami, J.; Hansen, M.; Porwit-MacDonald, A.; Jensen, B.A.; *et al.* Ultraviolet radiation exposure and risk of malignant lymphomas. *J. Natl. Cancer Inst.* **2005**, *97*, 199–209.

37. Grant, W.B. Lower vitamin-D production from solar ultraviolet-B irradiance may explain some differences in cancer survival rates. *J. Natl. Med. Assoc.* **2006**, *98*, 357–364.

38. Planta, M.B. Sunscreen and melanoma: Is our prevention message correct? *J. Am. Board Fam. Med.* **2011**, *24*, 735–739.

39. Pfeifer, M.; Begerow, B.; Minne, H.W. Vitamin D and muscle function. *Osteoporos. Int.* **2002**, *13*, 187–194.

40. Tague, S.E.; Clarke, G.L.; Winter, M.K.; McCarson, K.E.; Wright, D.E.; Smith, P.G. Vitamin D Deficiency Promotes Skeletal Muscle Hypersensitivity and Sensory Hyperinnervation. *J. Neurosci.* **2011**, *31*, 13728–13738.

41. Bhatty, S.A.; Shaikh, N.A.; Irfan, M.; Kashif, S.M.; Vaswani, A.S.; Sumbhai, A.; Gunpat. Vitamin D deficiency in fibromyalgia. *J. Pak. Med. Assoc.* **2010**, *60*, 949–951.

42. Clarke, N.M.; Page, J.E. Vitamin D deficiency: A paediatric orthopaedic perspective. *Curr. Opin. Pediatr.* **2012**, *24*, 46–49.

43. Von Kanel, R.; Muller-Hartmannsgruber, V.; Kokinogenis, G.; Egloff, N. Vitamin D and central hypersensitivity in patients with chronic pain. *Pain Med.* **2014**, doi:10.1111/pme.12454.

44. Le Goaziou, M.F.; Kellou, N.; Flori, M.; Perdrix, C.; Dupraz, C.; Bodier, E.; Souweine, G. Vitamin D supplementation for diffuse musculoskeletal pain: Results of a before-and-after study. *Eur. J. Gen. Pract.* **2014**, *20*, 3–9.

45. O'Brien, H.; Hershey, A.D.; Kabbouche, M.A. Prevalence of vitamin D among pediatric patients with recurrent headaches. *Headache* **2010**(Supplement 1), *50*, S23.
46. Nelson, K.B.; Richardson, A.K.; He, J.; Lateef, T.M.; Khoromi, S.; Merikangas, K.R. Headache and biomarkers predictive of vascular disease in a representative sample of US children. *Arch. Pediatr. Adolesc. Med.* **2010**, *164*, 358–362.
47. Tietjen, G.E.; Herial, N.A.; White, L.; Utley, C.; Kosmyna, J.M.; Khuder, S.A. Migraine and biomarkers of endothelial activation in young women. *Stroke* **2009**, *40*, 2977–2982.
48. Prakash, S.; Shah, N.D. Chronic tension-type headache with vitamin D deficiency: Casual or causal association? *Headache* **2009**, *49*, 1214–1222.
49. Eyles, D.W.; Smith, S.; Kinobe, R.; Hewison, M.; McGrath, J.J. Distribution of the vitamin D receptor and 1 alpha-hydroxylase in human brain. *J. Chem. Neuroanat.* **2005**, *29*, 21–30.
50. McCann, J.; Ames, B. Is there convincing biological or behavioral evidence linking vitamin D deficiency to brain dysfunction? *FASEB J.* **2008**, *22*, 982–1001.
51. Annweiler, C.; Schott, A.M.; Allali, G.; Bridenbaugh, S.A.; Kressig, R.W.; Allain, P.; Herrmann, F.R.; Beauchet, O. Association of vitamin D deficiency with cognitive impairment in older women: Cross-sectional study. *Neurology* **2010**, *74*, 27–32.
52. Gracious, B.L.; Finucane, T.L.; Friedman-Campbell, M.; Messing, S.; Parkhurst, M.N. Vitamin D deficiency and psychotic features in mentally ill adolescents: A cross-sectional study. *BMC Psychiatr.* **2012**, *12*, 38.
53. Humble, M.B.; Gustafsson, S.; Bejerot, S. Low serum levels of 25-hydroxyvitamin d(25OHD) among psychiatric out-patients in Sweden: Relations with season, age, ethnic origin andpsychiatric diagnosis. *J. Steroid Biochem. Mol. Biol.* **2010**, *121*, 467–470.
54. Högberg, G.; Gustafsson, S.A.; Hällström, T.; Gustafsson, T.; Klawitter, B.; Petersson, M. Depressed adolescents in a case-series were low in vitamin D and depression was ameliorated by vitamin D supplementation. *Acta Paediatr.* **2012**, *101*, 779–783.
55. CDC—Developmental Disabilities Monitoring Network Surveillance Year 2010 Principal Investigators. Prevalence of Autism Spectrum Disorder Among Children Aged 8 Years—Autism and Developmental Disabilities Monitoring Network, 11 Sites, United States, 2010. *MMWR Surveill. Summ.* **2014**, *63*, 1–21.
56. Kim, Y.S.; Leventhal, B.L.; Koh, Y.J.; Fombonne, E.; Laska, E.; Lim, E.C.; Cheon, K.A.; Kim, S.J.; Kim, Y.K.; Lee, H.; *et al.* Prevalence of autism spectrum disorders in atotal population sample. *Am. J. Psychiatr.* **2011**, *168*, 904–912.
57. Rossignol, D.A.; Frye, R.E. A review of research trends in physiological abnormalities inautism spectrum disorders: Immune dysregulation, inflammation, oxidative stress, mitochondrialdysfunction and environmental toxicant exposures. *Mol. Psychiatr.* **2012**, *17*, 389–401.
58. Patrick, R.P.; Ames, B.N. Vitamin D hormone regulates serotonin synthesis. Part 1: Relevance for autism. *FASEB J.* **2014**, *28*, 2398–2413.

59. Ashwood, P.; Krakowiak, P.; Hertz-Picciotto, I.; Hansen, R.; Pessah, I.; van de Water, J. Elevated plasma cytokines in autism spectrum disorders provide evidence of immune dysfunction and are associated with impaired behavioral outcome. *Brain Behav. Immun.* **2011**, *25*, 40–45.

60. Arnson, Y.; Itzhaky, D.; Mosseri, M.; Barak, V.; Tzur, B.; Agmon-Levin, N.; Amital, H. Vitamin D inflammatory cytokines and coronaryevents: A comprehensive review. *Clin. Rev. Allergy Immunol.* **2013**, *45*, 236–247.

61. Rose, S.; Melnyk, S.; Pavliv, O.; Bai, S.; Nick, T.G.; Frye, R.E.; James, S.J. Evidence of oxidative damage and inflammationassociated with low glutathione redox status in the autism brain. *Transl. Psychiatr.* **2012**, *2*, doi:10.1038/tp.2012.61.

62. Garcion, E.; Wion-Barbot, N.; Montero-Menei., C.N.; Berger, F.; Wion, D. New clues about vitamin D functions in the nervous system. *Trends Endocrinol. Metab.* **2002**, *13*, 100–105.

63. Christensen, J.; Grønborg, T.; Sørensen, M.; Schendel, D.; Parne, E.T.; Pedersen, L.H.; Vestergaard, M. Prenatal Valproate Exposure and Risk of Autism Spectrum Disorders and Childhood Autism. *JAMA* **2013**, *309*, 1696–1703.

64. Tomita, S.; Ohnishi, J.; Nakano, M.; Ichikawa, Y. The effects of anticonvulsant drugs on Vitamin D 3 -activating cytochrome P-450-linked monooxygenase systems. *J. Steroid Biochem. Mol. Biol.* **1991**, *39*, 479–485.

65. Deykin, E.Y.; MacMahon, B. The incidence of seizures among children with autisticsymptoms. *Am. J. Psychiatr.* **1979**, *136*, 1310–1312.

66. Holló, A.; Clemens, Z.; Kamondi, A.; Lakatos, P.; Szűcs, A. Correction of vitamin D deficiencyimproves seizure control in epilepsy: A pilot study. *Epilepsy Behav.* **2012**, *24*, 131133.

67. Numakawa, T.; Matsumoto, T.; Numakawa, Y.; Richards, M.; Yamawaki, S.; Kunugi1, H. Protective Action of Neurotrophic Factors and Estrogen against Oxidative Stress-Mediated Neurodegeneration. *J. Toxicol.* **2011**, 405194. doi:10.1155/2011/405194.

68. Maimburg, R.D.; Hammer-Bech, B.; Væth, M.; Møller-Madsen, B.; Olsen, J. Neonatal Jaundice, Autism, and OtherDisorders of Psychological Development. *Pediatrics* **2010**, *126*, 872–878.

69. Waldman, M.; Nicholson, S.; Adilov, N.; Williams, J. Autism prevalence and precipitation rates in California, Oregon, and Washington counties. *Arch. Pediatr. Adolesc. Med.* **2008**, *162*, 1026–1034.

70. Williams, J.G.; Higgins, J.P.; Brayne, C.E. Systematic review of prevalence studies of autismspectrum disorders. *Arch. Dis. Child.* **2006**, *91*, 8–15.

71. Cannell, J.J. Autism and vitamin D. *Med. Hypotheses* **2008**, *70*, 750–759.

72. Wei, S.Q.; Qi, H.P.; Luo, Z.C.; Fraser, W.D. Maternal vitamin D status and adverse pregnancy outcomes: A systematic review and meta-analysis. *J. Matern. Fetal. Neonatal Med.* **2013**, *26*, 889–899.

73. Jones, A.P.; Palmer, D.; Zhang, G.; Prescott, S.L. Cord blood 25-hydroxyvitamin D3 andallergic disease during infancy. *Pediatrics* **2012**, *130*, e1128–e1135.

74. Baïz, N.; Dargent-Molina, P.; Wark, J.D.; Souberbielle, J.C.; Annesi-Maesano, I. EDEN Mother-Child Cohort Study Group. Cord serum 25-hydroxyvitamin D and risk of early childhood transient wheezing and atopic dermatitis. *J. Allergy Clin. Immunol.* **2014**, *133*, 147–153.

75. Whitehouse, A.J.; Holt, B.J.; Serralha, M.; Holt, P.G.; Kusel, M.M.H.; Hart, P.H. Maternal serum vitamin D levels duringpregnancy and offspring neurocognitive development. *Pediatrics* **2012**, *129*, 485–493.

76. Schroth, R.J.; Lavelle, C.; Tate, R.; Bruce, S.; Billings, R.J.; Moffatt, M.E. Prenatal Vitamin D and Dental Caries in Infants. *Pediatrics* **2014**, 133:5 e1277-e1284.

77. Hollis, B.W.; Wagner, C.L. Vitamin D requirements during lactation: High-dose maternal supplementation as therapy to prevent hypovitaminosis D for both the mother and the nursinginfant. *Am. J. Clin. Nutr.* **2004**, *80*, 1752S–1758S.

78. Hollis, B.W.; Johnson, D.; Hulsey, T.C.; Ebeling, M.; Wagner, C.L. Vitamin D supplementation during pregnancy: Double-blind, randomized clinical trial of safety andeffectiveness. *J. Bone Miner. Res.* **2011**, *26*, 2341–2357.

79. Oberhelman, S.S.; Meekins, M.E.; Fischer, P.R.; Lee, B.R.; Singh, R.J.; Cha, S.S.; Gardner, B.M.; Pettifor, J.M.; Croghan, I.T.; Thacher, T.D. Maternal vitamin D supplementation to improve the vitamin D status of breast-fed infants: A randomized controlled trial. *Mayo Clin. Proc.* **2013**, *88*, 1378–1387.

80. Heaney, R.P.; Recker, R.R.; Grote, J.; Horst, R.L.; Armas, L.A. Vitamin D(3) is more potentthan vitamin D(2) in humans. *J. Clin. Endocrinol. Metab.* **2011**, *96*, E447–E452.

81. Mark, S.; Lambert, M.; Delvin, E.E.; O'Loughlin, J.; Tremblay, A.; Gray-Donald, K. Higher vitamin D intake is needed to achieve serum 25(OH)D levels greater than 50 nmol/l in Québec youth at high risk of obesity. *Eur. J. Clin. Nutr.* **2011**, *65*, 486–492.

82. Heaney, R.P.; Davies, K.M.; Chen, T.C.; Holick, M.F.; Barger-Lux, M.J. Human serum 25 hydroxycholecalciferol response to extended oral dosing with cholecalciferol. *Am. J. Clin. Nutr.* **2003**, *77*, 204–210.

83. Gallo, S.; Comeau, K.; Vanstone, C.; Agellon, S.; Sharma, A.; Jones, G.; L'Abbé, M.; Khamessan, A.; Rodd, C.; Weiler, H. Effect of different dosages of oral vitamin D supplementation on vitamin D status in healthy, breastfed infants: A randomized trial. *JAMA* **2013**, *309*, 1785–1792.

84. Cannell, J.J.; Vieth, R.; Willett, W.; Zasloff, M.; Hathcock, J.N.; White, J.H.; Tanumihardjo, S.A.; Larson-Meyer, D.E.; Bischoff-Ferrari, H.A.; Lamberg-Allardt, C.J.; *et al.* Cod liver oil, vitamin A toxicity, frequent respiratory infections, and the vitamin D deficiency epidemic. *Ann. Otol. Rhinol. Laryngol.* **2008**, *117*, 864–870.

85. Vieth, R.; Bischoff-Ferrari, H.; Boucher, B.J.; Dawson-Hughes, B.; Garland, C.F.; Heaney, R.P.; Holick, M.F.; Hollis, B.W.; Lamberg-Allardt, C.; McGrath, J.J.; *et al.* The urgent need to recommend an intake of vitamin D that is effective. *Am. J. Clin. Nutr.* **2007**, *85*, 649–650.

86. Grant, W.B.; Schwalfenberg, G.K.; Genuis, S.J.; Whiting, S.J. An estimate of the economic burden and premature deaths due to vitamin D deficiency in Canada. *Mol. Nutr. Food Res.* **2010**, *54*, 1172–1181.

87. Molinari, N.A.; Ortega-Sanchez, I.R.; Messonnier, M.L.; Thompson, W.W.; Wortley, P.M.; Weintraub, E.; Bridges, C.B. The annual impact of seasonal influenza in the US: Measuring disease burden and costs. *Vaccine* **2007**, *25*, 5086–5096.
88. Barnett, S.B.; Nurmagambetov, T.A. Costs of Asthma in the Unites States: 2002–2007. *J. Allergy Clin. Immunol.* **2011**, *127*, 145–152.
89. Fendrick, A.M.; Monto, A.S.; Nightengale, B.; Sarnes, M. The economic burden of noninfluenza related viral respiratory tract infection in the United States. *Arch. Intern. Med.* **2003**, *163*, 487–494.
90. Autism Speaks. Available online: http://www.autismspeaks.org (accessed on 1 September 2014).
91. National Institutes of Health. Available online: http://www.nhlbi.nih.gov/about/factpdf.htm (accessed on 1 September 2014).

Pediatric Integrative Medicine Approaches to Attention Deficit Hyperactivity Disorder (ADHD)

Anna Esparham, Randall G. Evans, Leigh E. Wagner and Jeanne A. Drisko

Abstract: Attention deficit hyperactivity disorder (ADHD) is the most common neuropsychiatric disorder in children and is increasing in prevalence. There has also been a related increase in prescribing stimulant medication despite some controversy whether ADHD medication makes a lasting difference in school performance or achievement. Families who are apprehensive about side effects and with concerns for efficacy of medication pursue integrative medicine as an alternative or adjunct to pharmacologic and cognitive behavioral treatment approaches. Integrative medicine incorporates evidence-based medicine, both conventional and complementary and alternative therapies, to deliver personalized care to the patient, emphasizing diet, nutrients, gut health, and environmental influences as a means to decrease symptoms associated with chronic disorders. Pediatric integrative medicine practitioners are increasing in number throughout the United States because of improvement in patient health outcomes. However, limited funding and poor research design interfere with generalizable treatment approaches utilizing integrative medicine. The use of research designs originally intended for drugs and procedures are not suitable for many integrative medicine approaches. This article serves to highlight integrative medicine approaches in use today for children with ADHD, including dietary therapies, nutritional supplements, environmental hygiene, and neurofeedback.

Reprinted from *Children*. Cite as: Esparham, A.; Evans, R.G.; Wagner, L.E.; Drisko, J.A. Pediatric Integrative Medicine Approaches to Attention Deficit Hyperactivity Disorder (ADHD). *Children* **2014**, *1*, 186–207.

1. Introduction

Attention deficit hyperactivity disorder (ADHD) is characterized as a psychiatric condition of heightened impulsivity, inattention, and hyperactivity [1]. ADHD is the most common neurodevelopment disorder in children, affecting approximately 11% of children between 4 and 17 years of age in the United States. Increased public awareness and escalation of inciting risk factors has been accompanied by an increased rate of ADHD diagnosis, along with a rise in medication use [2]. The definitive etiopathogenesis of ADHD remains elusive due to its complex, multifactorial nature. ADHD has strong genetic and environmental influences [3]. However, the increased prevalence of ADHD is likely due to genetics but rather these environmental factors. Nutritional status, oxidative stress, neurotransmitter and endocrine dysregulation, neurological abnormalities in fronto-striatal and basal ganglia network, history of physical and emotional trauma, and environmental toxicity have all been implicated in ADHD [4–9]. In order to identify the most appropriate treatment, healthcare providers should identify these risk factors with a thorough evaluation of the child with ADHD.

It is crucial that children with ADHD are treated appropriately as they can develop significant psychosocial, educational, and neuropsychological impairment [10]. They are also at risk for not achieving their highest potential in education and employment as adults [11]. Behavioral therapy and medications are central to the management of ADHD, resulting in greater improvements in academic performance, reduction of behavioral problems, and higher parental satisfaction [12,13]. Limited access to mental health professionals interferes with the utility of psychosocial therapy. Only one-third of youths treated for ADHD received both psychosocial therapy and medications, and less than 10% received psychosocial interventions alone [14]. Children with ADHD also exhibit several comorbid disorders, resulting in decreased response to treatment.

Medication for ADHD is associated with its own set of problems. Twenty to 35% of patients with ADHD do not respond to medication. In addition, medications have significant adverse effects with the most common side effects including delayed onset of sleep and decreased appetite both known to potentiate symptoms of ADHD. This results in discontinuation of medication as a result of side effects and the parents' perception that the medication is ineffective; another factor in medication cessation is the cost burden for families [15,16]. Thus, families are seeking different approaches to treatment, including complementary and alternative therapies (CAM).

The 2007 National Health Interview Survey discovered that approximately 12 percent of children in the United States have used or been given a CAM therapy [17]. More than 50% of Children with ADHD have been reported to use CAM therapies, but only 11% of parents discuss CAM therapies with their child's physician [18]. As physicians are reluctant to incorporate CAM therapies because they question their scientific efficacy, there is continued need for research and education of these CAM therapies. There is a subset of pediatricians who utilize both conventional and CAM therapies, a field known as integrative medicine, in order to improve outcomes in children with ADHD. Integrative medicine incorporates evidence-based medicine, both conventional and complementary and alternative therapies, to deliver personalized care to the patient, emphasizing diet, nutrients, gut health, and environmental influences as a means to decrease symptoms associated with chronic disorders. Pediatric integrative medicine (PIM) is a fairly new subspecialty and is defined as a relationship-centered practice that utilizes the best evidence in therapeutic approaches to achieve optimal health for children [19]. This review is designed to educate healthcare professionals on a PIM approach to ADHD to help initiate discussions of CAM use with patients and families.

2. Diet

What children eat has a profound effect on their health. Although controversial, dietary therapies have been suggested to play a major role in ADHD and should be considered in the evaluation and management of children with ADHD [20–22]. Nutritional deficiencies from a "Western" diet, food insecurity, artificial food additives and dyes, and food sensitivities and allergies have been implicated in ADHD [23–28]. Most research related to dietary constituents has focused on restricted elimination diets (RED), sugar restriction, and artificial food color exclusion diets in the treatment of ADHD. A research review identified that dietary constituents can significantly worsen ADHD symptoms in 17 of 23 controlled studies [29]. As oxidative stress, or inflammation, is an underlying risk factor in ADHD, modulation of systemic inflammation through nutrition may have potential in decreasing symptoms of youth with ADHD [30]. A Western diet that is high in omega-6 fatty acids, sodium, and sugar intake can induce inflammation, promoting upregulation of pro-inflammatory TH17 cells, cytokines, and IL-10 [31].

2.1. Restricted Elimination Diet (RED)

Although adherence is difficult and time consuming, RED has been shown to benefit children with ADHD. The Impact of Nutrition in Children with ADHD (INCA) was a double-blind crossover research study that showed children ages 4–8 years old improve on the abbreviated Conners' scale by 11.6 after being placed on a tailored RED for five weeks [26]. Furthermore, 63% of the children relapsed with ADHD symptoms after a food challenge. The INCA study found that IgG blood levels did not correlate with ADHD symptoms. This study was well designed with good methodology, large sample size, and correlation with IgG food antigen blood tests. In addition, the diets were specifically tailored to each participant, which helped improve adherence [26]. Due to the recurrence of ADHD symptoms after a five-week RED, more research trials need to investigate how long children with ADHD need to stay on a RED in order to prevent recurrence of symptoms during a food challenge. Some review articles evaluating RED to treat ADHD have discussed that the diet may only influence some aspects of ADHD, such as behavior, and that it should only be done in a select few and for a short period of time of 2–3 weeks [20]. However, antibodies have a half-life between 22–96 days and more improvement in symptoms may be seen with a three-month RED [32]. After approximately 3–6 months, those children who show improvements in behavior and a decrease in ADHD symptoms on RED should introduce one food at a time every one to two weeks until offending foods or food items are identified.

2.2. Junk Food Diet

PIM physicians begin with a whole foods, non-processed diet for children with ADHD [33]. Children with ADHD symptoms are at increased risk for becoming obese in adolescence and this is correlated with poor dietary choices and physical inactivity [34]. Children today are exposed to aggressive advertising for highly processed and sugary foods, influencing their eating behaviors [35]. A diet high in processed foods and sugar, otherwise known as "junk food," has been studied in children with ADHD, though very little evidence has demonstrated associations. One study demonstrated a modest association between children who ate junk food and hyperactivity symptoms, but attenuated after adjustment for confounders [36]. In two separate research studies, sucrose was associated with an increase in motor activity and was shown to reduce attention in children with ADHD, but not in normal children [37,38]. There has been little evidence to support an association between sugar intake and behavioral problems [38,39]. These research studies have not found any association on sugar consumption and ADHD, but cannot rule out a small effect on subsets of children with ADHD [38,39]. In addition, these research studies used artificial sweeteners as the placebo group. This may confound the results because artificial sweeteners have been implicated in neuropsychiatric dysfunction [40,41]. These few research studies also evaluated response to acute effects of sugar consumption, but did not evaluate chronic effects. Further research should evaluate not just sucrose consumption, but excess and chronic carbohydrate consumption and its effect on ADHD symptomology as providers report improvements in behavior with a whole foods diet.

3. Gluten-Related Disorders

Gluten-free diets have been implemented for children with neuropsychiatric disorders, including autism and ADHD [7]. Gluten-related disorders, such as celiac disease (CD) and gluten sensitivity, may be associated with ADHD. CD results in gluten-triggered autoimmune intestinal villi destruction in genetically susceptible individuals. Non-celiac gluten sensitivity (NCGS) is a condition in which gluten ingestion leads to morphological or symptomatic manifestations despite the absence of CD. NCGS and CD are triggered by the ingestion of gluten, or more specifically gliadin, the protein components of wheat, rye, and barley. Exposure results in a variable degree of intestinal damage that can induce intestinal permeability, resulting in extra-intestinal manifestations. These extra-intestinal symptoms can masquerade as behavioral and psychiatric disorders.

In the 1950s and 1960s, physicians first began reporting neurologic and psychotic symptoms in patients with CD [42]. There has been emerging evidence to show that individuals with gluten-related disorders, such as CD and NCGS, have neurologic, psychiatric and mood disorders [43–45]. Gluten-free diets are becoming widely accepted in the United States [46]. Furthermore, avoiding gluten is common among non-CD children who exhibit nonspecific behavioral and gastrointestinal symptoms [47]. However, there are few research trials done specifically in regards to gluten and its association with ADHD. Dr. Helmut Neiderhofer, MD, PhD and Dr. Klaus Pittschieler, MD demonstrated an increased prevalence of CD in ADHD patients and also noted improved ADHD symptoms after implementation of gluten-free diet in children with CD [48,49]. Inattention has been found to be associated in children with CD compared to healthy children, though a conflicting study by Gungor et al. did not show any association between CD and ADHD [48,50, 51]. However, it still remains that gluten withdrawal in neuropsychiatric disorders results in improved mood, focus and attention, as well as a decrease in disruptive behaviors [52,53].

The mechanism of action behind gluten's effect on neuropsychiatric symptoms is still inconclusive, but gastrointestinal immune dysregulation can lead to chronic pro-inflammatory immune dysregulation. This chronic inflammation may be one of the underlying links in the development of ADHD [7,30]. It is also hypothesized that gluten can induce gastrointestinal inflammation, thereby limiting absorption of nutrients and disrupting neurotransmitter metabolism [54].

Despite conflicting evidence of CD and its association with ADHD, clinicians should focus on a broad array of symptoms when evaluating children with ADHD, including both gastrointestinal and neuropsychiatric symptoms to rule out CD or NCGS as an exacerbating condition. Screening for and diagnosing CD and NCGS remains a challenge. A research trial assessed the usefulness of screening for CD when children presented with common CD symptoms (e.g., poor appetite, stomach ache, nausea, bloating, tiredness, hard stools, loose stools and lactose intolerance) [55]. The study results showed that screening children based on only these symptoms did not discriminate

60

between undiagnosed children with CD-associated symptoms and asymptomatic CD children. Determination of NCGS is difficult due to lack of consensus on specific biomarkers, as opposed to CD. Positive effects after gluten withdrawal and return of symptoms with gluten challenge are the main diagnostic criteria [56–58]. In most patients with CD and NCGS, the gastrointestinal and extra-intestinal symptoms will reverse on a gluten-free diet [59].

If the decision is made to choose a gluten-free diet, this should be implemented by a team of healthcare professionals, including a trained dietitian, as it is easy to replace wheat/gluten-containing products with gluten-free products high in refined carbohydrates, but low in fiber and nutrients. And if a gluten-free diet is not a good fit, a whole foods diet rich in fresh unprocessed foods is ideal. Most patients with ADHD would benefit from a whole foods diet.

4. Micronutrients

The value of nutrition is increasingly becoming recognized as a means for achieving optimal health, as poor diet and nutritional intake are implicated in chronic disorders [60]. Most studies in ADHD and nutrients have focused on polyunsaturated fatty acids and a few minerals, including magnesium, zinc and iron. However, there are many more micronutrients than those that have been predominantly studied. Micronutrients are utilized as cofactors in enzymatic reactions and play a large role in metabolism, neurotransmission, cognitive function, immune function, and detoxification [61,62]. Instead of looking at only a few micronutrients, a comprehensive but focused nutrient panel may be done for those children who have failed conventional treatment approaches or for those families who are exploring other options besides medication. A comprehensive micronutrient panel may include vitamins, minerals, fatty acids, and amino acids, as the quality of our nutrient supply from food has declined [63].

4.1. Zinc

Zinc is known to a play a role in neuropsychiatric disorders and is a micronutrient recognized as participating in metabolism relevant to neurotransmitters, hormones, nutrients, and immune function [64,65]. It also contributes to the structure and function of the brain, forming neural pathways affecting neurotransmission [66]. Zinc deficiency can thus have a significant impact on attention, motor activity, cognition, and behavior. Approximately 12%–66% of the world's population is at risk of zinc deficiency, and is seen especially in children with ADHD who are vulnerable to poor zinc status [67,68]. Although a Cochrane review of 13 randomized trials did not demonstrate a positive effect of zinc supplementation on mental and motor development, there have been several review articles discussing positive improvements in ADHD symptoms with zinc supplementation [69–71]. There have been three positive randomized controlled studies on zinc supplementation *versus* placebo in children with ADHD. Bilici *et al.* demonstrated that zinc decreased motor activity and improved impulsivity, but did not increase attention [72]. Akhondzadeh's *et al.* showed improvement in total ADHD scores with the addition of elemental zinc 13 mg/day to methylphenidate 1 mg/kg/day *versus* placebo and methylphenidate [73]. In a study by Arnold and colleagues, children on zinc supplementation were able to lower their dose of amphetamine, though zinc did not improve inattention or other ADHD symptoms more than placebo [74]. There is encouraging support for zinc supplementation in a subset of children with ADHD, depending on symptoms and if used in combination with stimulants.

4.2. Iron

Iron status is commonly evaluated in children with neuropsychiatric disorders likely due to its role as a cofactor in monoaminergic neurotransmitter metabolism [75]. Research has suggested that iron status should be investigated in order to optimize treatment outcomes with stimulant medication [76]. With the prevalence of sleep disturbance in ADHD, Cortese and colleagues found that serum ferritin levels below 45 microg/L may provide evidence to supplement iron in those children with sleep disorder [77]. There are some significant and non-significant associations between serum ferritin levels and ADHD symptoms, but most of these studies focused on serum ferritin levels without other iron indices. As inflammation and oxidative stress have been implicated in the etiopathogenesis of ADHD, serum ferritin is an inflammatory marker when elevated, which may complicate its evaluation. In addition, excess inflammation and low levels of glutathione, the main body's detoxifier and antioxidant, can result in iron dysregulation [78]. It may be worthwhile then to evaluate a complete blood count with differential and serum ferritin with iron panel to help guide management in children with ADHD, especially when associated with more complex symptoms, including sleep disturbance.

4.3. Vitamin B6

Insufficient Vitamin B6, also known as pyridoxine or pyridoxal-5-phosphate, affects metabolism of polyunsaturated fatty acids, hemoglobin synthesis, and neurotransmission [62]. It was later found that pyridoxine is a cofactor in neurotransmitter metabolism including serotonin, glutamate/GABA, and dopamine. Because pyridoxine has a positive effect on children with ADHD, it is recommended to supplement in order to regulate and normalize ADHD behaviors [79]. In fact, a pharmaceutical medication, metadoxine, is an ion-pair salt of pyridoxine that has shown to improve inattentive symptoms, but only studied in the adult population with ADHD [80]. By regulating neurotransmission, vitamin B6 may improve executive function and symptoms of ADHD. Vitamin B6 is generally safe without serious side effects and should be considered in the evaluation of children with ADHD.

4.4. Magnesium

Magnesium is the fourth most abundant mineral and is involved as a cofactor in over 300 enzymatic reactions in the body, including fatty acid, glucose and energy metabolism [62]. Some of these metabolic processes play a vital role in neuronal function and neurotransmitter metabolism [81]. Some investigators have proposed magnesium supplementation is advantageous for ADHD symptoms [33,82–84]. Magnesium acts as a neuroprotectant from excessive excitatory neurotransmitters, such as glutamate [85]. Several studies have found low erythrocyte or RBC (red blood cell) magnesium in children with ADHD [68,82,84,86]. Although a systematic review of magnesium therapy for treating ADHD did not show a significant improvement in symptoms, most of these studies had methodological limitations, including many that were not double-blind randomized controlled clinical trials, and magnesium was measured inappropriately [87]. Therefore, RBC magnesium, a sensitive biomarker for magnesium deficiency, should be incorporated into future clinical trials and may be important in the work-up for children with ADHD. Appropriate magnesium supplementation may be a useful adjunct for children on stimulant medication.

4.5. Polyunsaturated Fatty Acids

Polyunsaturated fatty acid (PUFAs) disturbance has also been implicated in ADHD, as they are necessary for nerve cell membrane fluidity and neuronal function to support neurotransmission. However, the typical American diet contains an imbalance of omega-6 to omega-3 PUFAs. An elevated Omega-6 to Omega-3 ratio is implicated in inflammation [88,89]. Omega-6 fatty acids derived from canola oil, corn oil, soybean oil, and other vegetable fats are inflammatory in nature as they metabolize downstream to arachidonic acid. Arachidonic acid subsequently produces inflammatory prostaglandins and leukotrienes. Gamma-linolenic acid, an n-6 fatty acid, is the exception to the rule which has been shown to be anti-inflammatory in nature [90]. Limiting restaurant and take-out food is also important in balancing PUFAs to reduce inflammatory omega-6 fats because of the prevalence of use and the tendency to damage fats during high heat cooking conditions.

Omega-3 fatty acids, found in flaxseeds, chia seeds, and fatty fish, metabolize downstream to anti-inflammatory prostaglandins and leukotrienes [89,91]. With the increased prevalence of farmed fish, there are less omega-3s produced than are found in their wild counterparts [92]. Dr. Susan Carlson, PhD and her team have found that DHA, an n-3 fatty acid, is essential in neurocognitive development of children. Her research suggests that DHA should be supplemented throughout the lifecycle due to its importance in neuropsychiatric disorders [93].

Practitioners, including dietitians, can help guide families of children with ADHD to increase balanced portions of healthy fats and decrease the inflammatory fats. As research has identified elevated inflammatory markers in children and adolescents with ADHD, maintaining a healthy omega-6 to omega-3 ratio with a diet containing healthy balances of PUFAs, saturated fats, and phospholipids may be a promising integrative medicine approach to treatment of ADHD [94].

However, some reports using placebo-controlled randomized controlled trials (RCTs) evaluating PUFAs efficacy in treating ADHD differ in conclusions [95–99]. Research studies using PUFAs for ADHD that did not reach statistical significance may likely be due to the different combinations, doses, and frequency of PUFA mixes (ALA/LA/EPA/DHA/GLA ratios), in addition to using a placebo with nutritional properties, such as olive oil and vitamin C [97–100]. The Cochrane review demonstrated that a subgroup of children with ADHD did show improvement with EPA, DHA, and a small amount of GLA [101]. A meta-analysis also demonstrated an effect size of 0.31 for omega-3 fatty acid supplements [95]. When compared to methylphenidate with an effect size of 0.78, Omega-3 fatty acids as a single supplement are approximately 40% as effective as methylphenidate [95,102]. Also, most of these studies did not evaluate phospholipids, such as phosphatidylcholine, essential in neurodevelopment and has been shown to enhance the effect of omega-3 supplements [103].

In clinical practice, evaluation of fatty acids using a comprehensive serum fatty acid panel or RBC fatty acid panel to guide supplementation may be an effective strategy for optimizing treatment outcomes. Fatty acid synthesis and metabolism also involves several other micronutrients as cofactors for the desaturase and elongase enzymes and these may be evaluated by laboratory testing [62]. Individuals vary in need depending on dietary intake and metabolism of fatty acids. PUFAs and associated micronutrient supplementation should be tailored to the individual using guidelines as reports of adverse events exist in the research literature, such as over supplementation of omega-3 fatty acids may increase bleeding time [104]. However, following a healthcare practitioner's advice on adding PUFAs and monounsaturated fats from fish, flax and chia seeds, nuts, avocado, extra virgin olive oil, and healthy saturated fats from coconut oil is likely advantageous to a child with ADHD.

4.6. Carnitine

Carnitine is a fatty acid transporter that transfers long chain fatty acids across mitochondrial membrane for beta-oxidation. Acetyl L-carnitine is an abundant short chain ester of carnitine, which has an effect on brain metabolism and neurotransmission, specifically the cholinergic and dopaminergic pathways [105,106]. Three placebo-controlled trials on carnitine supplementation in participants with ADHD from 2002 to current have been conducted [107–109]. However, only one of these small trials showed an improvement after supplementation with carnitine in attention and decrease in aggression in boys with ADHD [108]. Two studies did not demonstrate a significant benefit, but one study found that it did attenuate the side effects of irritability and headaches of methylphenidate [106,108]. However, these two studies did not distinguish between subtypes of ADHD and did not evaluate carnitine levels at baseline and post-treatment. It has to be considered that these children may not have any nutritional need for carnitine supplementation. Carnitine needs further evaluation in future research studies to adequately assess effects in children with ADHD.

4.7. Vitamin D

Vitamin D is now implicated in ADHD [110]. Vitamin D is essential for normal brain development and regulates both the innate and adaptive immune system enhancing neuroprotective mechanisms against inflammation [111,112]. A case-control study in Qatar of 1,331 children ages 5–18 years old demonstrated a higher prevalence of vitamin D deficiency in the ADHD children compared to controls [110]. In 2001, a study done by Taylor *et al.* surveyed parents to compare symptoms of their child with ADHD when they were engaging in leisure activities in a windowless room *versus* in an outdoor setting where natural production of vitamin D will occur. The survey results demonstrated that the outdoor setting was more likely to be chosen by parents to reduce inattentive symptoms [113]. Sunlight and vitamin D may be considered a major participant in improving certain symptoms of ADHD and a decrease in outdoor activity with less sunlight exposure may have contributed to the higher prevalence of vitamin D deficiency in children with

ADHD. Supplementing children with vitamin D guided by lab results may be a safe and effective strategy to help improve symptoms.

4.8. Iodine

For women of childbearing age, iodine insufficiency is approximately 15% in the United States. Pregnant women in the United States are at slight risk of iodine insufficiency especially in the first trimester [114. Iodine deficiency can be measured by a low urine iodine of less than 100 microg/L [62] In women who are planning to become pregnant and are found to be deficient, supplemental iodine may needed to optimize iodine status to ensure healthy cognitive development of the fetus. In addition, psychomotor development and cognitive performance declines in children with iodine insufficiency and iodine status should regularly be evaluated in children with ADHD. A synthesis of the research on iodine deficiency and its relationship to other disease processes other than thyroid disorders has associated iodine deficiency with the occurrence of ADHD [115].

The recommended daily allowance of up to 150 micrograms/day is meant to prevent goiter or thyroid disease [115]. It should be considered that this is not the optimal dose for all individuals who have different metabolic needs and thyroid function. Serial urine iodine measurements should be done until iodine status normalization. More studies are needed to evaluate iodine status and replacement strategies in children with ADHD, as subnormal levels of iodine can have an impact on a child's ability to focus and concentrate on school tasks.

5. Gut Microbiome

Humans have 100 trillion microbes residing in the gastrointestinal tract, some of which may be commensal, while others are pathologic [116]. Consumption of these healthy commensal microbes known as probiotics, have been shown to modulate brain activity [117]. Research has shown that there is a gut microbiome–mind–body continuum in which the enteric microbiota interact with the neuroendocrine system [118]. The gut microbiome essentially has its own nervous system, as it produces neuroendocrine hormones that transmit information across the microbiome [119]. There is increasing evidence that gut bacteria can modulate mood and behavior via the gut–brain axis [120]. Most of these studies have been done in germ-free animals who exhibited changes in mental status and behavior when exposed to pathogenic bacteria, probiotics, or antibiotics. The establishment of a healthy gut microbiome takes place early in development. Infants who were born via cesarean delivery had less microflora in their intestinal tract than those infants born by vaginal delivery [121]. This is consistent with Cesarean birth as a major risk factor of ADHD [122]. Additional evaluation of gut microbiome in ADHD children is therefore warranted.

As part of the practice at University of Kansas Pediatric Integrative Medicine, evaluation of children with neurodevelopment and mood disorders includes stool analysis for intestinal dysbiosis. Medications, such as antibiotics, can disrupt the gut microbiome by reducing diversity and allowing overgrowth of some pathogenic microorganisms [123]. Gut microbiota, such as Candida, can invade the intestine as a pathogen and may lead to deterioration in ADHD symptoms [124]. A Western diet, even in a short-term period, can alter the gut microbiome, again demonstrating the importance of diet and nutrition as a valuable therapy in ADHD [125]. The evidence surrounding the association with healthy gut microbiome and its relationship with psychiatric and behavioral disorders is increasing. This will present new opportunities for interventions with pre- and probiotics, as they are already in common use among families who use integrative therapies.

6. Environmental Toxicity

Industry produces over 83,000 chemicals greater than one million pounds per year with little information about the potential effects on neurodevelopment [126,127]. Approximately 1,000 of these chemicals can affect the nervous system, and at least 200 of these are known neurotoxins [128]. Children are highly susceptible to environmental chemicals, especially during preconception and as an infant through breast milk. Exposures to chemicals can alter epigenetic programming, leading to disruptions in neurodevelopment [129]. Recent research studies have now shown that transgenerational changes may even occur when grandparents of the child are exposed to environmental chemicals. Most testing has been done on animals, but these research studies still provide sufficient results to indicate toxic effects in human neurodevelopment [129]. Children also have a larger body surface area with higher respirations leaving them more susceptible to even low-dose chemical exposures through breathing, dermal contact, and food compared to adults. In a cohort of 607 children aged 7–11 years, investigators found an association between low-level prenatal organochlorine exposure via cord blood and ADHD behaviors in childhood [130]. The risk of ADHD-like behaviors in these children increased by 26% to 92%, according to the level of organochlorine exposure [130]. Organochlorines, including polychlorinated biphenyls (PCBs), are environmentally persistent chemicals that cross the placenta and have been shown to alter neurodevelopment [131]. Organophosphates, widely used as pesticides, remain another important avenue for neurodevelopment toxicity in children [132]. Urinary metabolites of organophosphates were obtained from the National Health and Nutrition Examination Survey (NHANES) on 1,139 children. The analyses demonstrated that the children with higher levels of exposure to organophosphates were more likely to have a diagnosis of ADHD [132]. In children, fruits and vegetables may be the most important source of chronic pesticide exposure [133]. This was demonstrated in a study by comparing organic *vs.* conventional diets in children, attesting that organic diets have a protective effect against exposure to organophosphate pesticides [133]. Recommendations to avoid or wash thoroughly the "dirty dozen" conventional produce and eating more of the "Clean 15" may be a beneficial nutritional approach for children with ADHD [134,135].

In addition to obtaining a thorough diet history in patients with ADHD, environmental exposure history needs to be evaluated and addressed. Some families may have a history of using herbicides, insecticides, chemicals including cleaning supplies, and volatile organic compounds, such as air fresheners in their homes. Education is of utmost importance to keep chemical exposure at a minimum. In fact, healthy housing initiatives are gaining popularity among medical communities to help control and prevent chronic disease in children. Advising families to opt for more natural solutions, such as "green" cleaning products that do not contain toxic industrial chemicals and using sticky traps for pests may be healthier alternatives. Limiting plastic products, such as plastic water bottles and microwaveable plastic containers, may also protect against ADHD, as there are positive associations between ADHD and bisphenol A (BPA) and phthalates commonly found in plastics [136].

Of the heavy metals, lead toxicity has been associated with ADHD and other neuropsychiatric disorders. It is well known that lead can cause cognitive impairment and attention dysregulation [137,138]. In a study of 236 children diagnosed with ADHD, low levels of lead exposure demonstrated an increased risk of ADHD [137]. In 2012, the Advisory Committee on Childhood Lead Poisoning Prevention of the Centers for Disease Control and Prevention (CDC) issued updated and stricter guidelines due to long-term effects on neurodevelopment of even low-level lead exposure [138]. Increasing the awareness of healthcare providers, families and the community to environmental chemical and heavy metal exposures is vital to the adjunctive management of these children with ADHD.

7. Neurofeedback

One of the most promising treatments in ADHD is neurofeedback, which is an EEG-based form of biofeedback. Neurofeedback is a safe, non-invasive therapy that restores the brain's ability to function through altering brain wave patterns by operant conditioning [139]. The individual can achieve self-regulation by responding to feedback from real-time audio-visual information. Quantitative EEG studies suggest that children with ADHD exhibit slower brainwave patterns in brain regions, such as the prefrontal cortex, associated with attention and cognitive executive function which is consistent with single photon emission computed tomography (SPECT) and positron emission tomography (PET) studies where decreased metabolism in prefrontal regions is identified [140]. In 1976, Lubar and Shouse were the first to report positive changes in a hyperkinetic child after training the Sensorimotor EEG rhythm (SMR: 12–14 Hz) [141]. Lubar then went on to develop protocols that inhibited theta (slow waves) and rewarded beta (fast waves involved in focus and attention). The FDA announced in July 2013 the approval of diagnosing ADHD by measuring the theta/beta ratio which has been shown to be higher in children with ADHD than normal children [142]. However, excessive theta/beta ratio may only characterize a subgroup of ADHD, approximately 26% of pediatric ADHD patients, compared with 2.5% in healthy controls [143–145]. Some studies have concluded that responders to stimulant medications have an initial excess of slow wave (theta) activity. After treatment with stimulant medication, increased beta waves and reduced theta waves result [146]. Stimulant medications may work not only through regulating neurotransmission, but also by affecting brain waves. A quantitative EEG (*i.e.*, brain map), utilized as initial baseline testing of brainwaves, should also be considered in future research studies as an evaluation tool for identifying responders and non-responders to ADHD medication [147]. Other identified EEG phenotypes of ADHD have also been reported including, excess beta, excess alpha, low alpha peak frequency and hypercoherence [143].

In 2004, Slow Cortical Potential (SCP) neurofeedback was found to improve ADHD symptoms [148]. SCP neurofeedback rewards changes in the polarity of the EEG and was initially used to treat epilepsy [149]. SCP neurofeedback enhances regulation of attention through slowly balancing cortical activation and inhibition. Children with ADHD have a significant reduction in the ability to regulate SCPs. In a RCT trial by Gevensleben and his colleagues, 102 children with

ADHD participated in neurofeedback and the control group participated in computerized attention skills training. The neurofeedback group completed one block of 18 theta/beta training sessions and one block of 18 SCP training sessions. At a six-month follow-up, reductions in inattention and hyperactivity/impulsivity were about 25%–35% in the neurofeedback group compared to 10%–15% in the control group with a group effect of 4.72 for inattention and 3.45 for hyperactivity/impulsivity [150]. SCP neurofeedback is recognized as an efficacious treatment for ADHD, though future studies still need to identify a sham control and improve efforts to blind participants, parents, teachers, and technicians [151].

A recent RCT research study on 23 children with ADHD carried out 40 sessions of theta/beta training sessions or methylphenidate and compared the two therapies with a six-month follow-up. Although this study had a limitation of small sample size, and 8 out of 12 participants in the neurofeedback group started medication, neurofeedback training was comparable to methylphenidate in reducing ADHD primary symptoms and associated functional impairment. Academic performance significantly improved in the neurofeedback group compared to the group receiving methylphenidate [152].

Despite promising results among research studies and anecdotal evidence, neurofeedback treatment is not yet accepted as a standard therapy for children with ADHD. This is possibly due to limitations of scientific research in neurofeedback accompanied by the difficulty in conducting a well-designed randomized controlled trial. Sham neurofeedback groups are designed as control groups in neurofeedback research. However, attention by neurofeedback technicians may result in positive gains in the control group. Subjective treatment effects can threaten the validity of neurofeedback research and these include participants, parents, and teachers' expectations of beneficial outcomes, provider training and experience, environmental stressors surrounding the participant, and participants' engagement during training. In a research update by Loo and Makeig, although the evidence is growing for scientific quality of research in neurofeedback, more research is needed before neurofeedback can be recommended as a first-line, stand-alone treatment modality [143].

In addition, neurofeedback participants must be encouraged to strive toward mastering engagement and regulation [153]. Participants should be rewarded during neurofeedback therapy to further enhance operant conditioning learning. This raises a question about the feasibility of conducting double-blind placebo-controlled trials. Neurofeedback protocols should be guided based on the individual's baseline qualitative EEG (QEEG), as one child with ADHD may have a different QEEG than another child with ADHD. Hence, protocols used in research may not be applicable to the individual and therefore, neurofeedback, may need to be considered a personalized therapy for improved clinical outcomes in ADHD.

8. Future Research

Some of the research related to integrative therapies for children with ADHD has shown mixed results. Of the integrative medicine approaches, the best evidence is for restricted elimination diets, neurofeedback, omega-3 fatty acid supplements, vitamin B6, and zinc. More rigorous and applicable research trials need to be funded in order to identify effective integrative therapies as standard practice. Some researchers suspect the "placebo effect" is responsible for the improvement seen with some integrative therapies. On the other hand, the "placebo effect" can account for perceived improvement from medications and other conventional therapies.

Unfortunately, research is limited in integrative medicine approaches to ADHD. This may be due to funding of and difficulty in designing randomized controlled trials (RCTs), considered the gold standard of evaluating treatment interventions. Evidence-based medicine was initially designed for drugs and procedures, but has been applied to nutrients and other integrative therapies. The high internal validity of RCTs can impede its external validity, meaning that it may not be generalizable to real-life situations, and applicability to the individual may be questionable. Hence, RCTs may not be the best tool to evaluate integrative therapies compared to other types of study designs, such as a pragmatic study design. For example, a single neurofeedback protocol for the general population may not be appropriate for the individual due to differences in brainwaves, genetics, diet, and environmental conditions. Pragmatic trials may be more efficacious in assessing integrative therapeutic approaches in real-life settings, compared to the controlled environments that do not take place outside of the research trial [154]. Evidence-based medicine was initially designed for drugs and procedures, but has been applied to nutrients. To effectively evaluate nutrients, research trials need to be redesigned to account for the difference between drugs and nutrients [155]. The best evidence, however, for an integrative intervention may be from outcome trials.

9. Conclusions

With adverse effects of and poor outcomes in long-term safety studies evaluating ADHD medications, more families are turning to integrative modalities to help decrease symptoms and improve quality of life in their children with ADHD. Integrative medicine may provide an alternative approach to treating ADHD, especially for those classified as non-responders. Because a significant percentage of the population with ADHD is classified as non-responsive, integrative medicine approaches to ADHD have gained popularity among families and practitioners. Because research is limited and outcomes show conflicting results, it is difficult for conventional practitioners to advise ADHD patients and their families when questions about integrative therapies arise. Partnering with an experienced pediatrician of integrative medicine may provide an outlet for treatment options and a trusted source for unanswered questions. Since the numbers of pediatricians of integrative medicine are growing, there is an expanding workforce that can provide guidance to conventional practitioners and families and help with design of future clinical trials in ADHD. Healthcare providers need to be aware of integrative modalities in use by families of children with ADHD in order to keep open communication when providing advice on possible benefits and/or limitations based on current research. This will help foster improved communication between families and patients with ADHD and their practitioners.

Acknowledgments

No grants or funds were received for this review article.

Author Contributions

Anna Esparham, MD is the lead author of this review article with expertise in pediatric integrative medicine for children with ADHD. She is a board-certified pediatrician with a fellowship in integrative medicine at the University of Kansas Medical Center Integrative Medicine (KU IM). She provided contributions to this article through organizing, directing, writing and editing the major sections.

Randall Evans, MS, RD, LD and is a dietitian at KU IM with a Master's degree in dietetics and integrative medicine with extensive experience in dietary interventions for parents of children with ADHD to decrease excess sugar and increase whole foods for lifestyle change. He provided guidance on the section of "junk food diets" with attention to gaps in the scientific literature.

Leigh Wagner, MS, RD, LD is a dietitian at KU IM with a Master's in dietetics and integrative medicine with experience in restricted elimination diets (RED) for young children with ADHD. She advised on the section of RED through synthesis of the most compelling scientific evidence.

Jeanne Drisko, MD is the founder and program director of KU IM with board certification in neurofeedback. She contributed to this paper through writing and advising the review of the entire manuscript.

Conflicts of Interest

The authors declare no conflict of interest.

References

1. American Psychiatric Association. *DSM-5 Fact Sheet: Attention Deficit/Hyperactivity Disorder*; American Psychiatric Publishing: Arlington, VA, USA, 2013.
2. Centers for Disease Control and Prevention (2013): Attention-Deficit/Hyperactivity Disorder. Available online: http://www.cdc.gov/ncbddd/adhd/data.html (accessed on 17 March, 2014).
3. Lehn, H.; Derks, E.M.; Hudziak, J.J.; Heutink, P.; van Beijsterveldt, T.C.; Boomsma, D.I. Attention problems and attention-deficit/hyperactivity disorder in discordant and concordant monozygotic twins: Evidence of environmental mediators. *J. Am. Acad. Child Adolesc. Psychiatry* 2007, *46*, 83–91.
4. Froehlich, T.E.; Loe, I.M.; Gilman, R.C. Update on Environmental Risk Factors for Attention-Deficit/Hyperactivity Disorder. *Curr. Psychiatry Rep.* 2012, *13*, 333–344.
5. Golmirzaei, J.; Namazi, S.; Amiri, S.; Zare, S.; Rastikerdar, N.; Hesam, A.A.; Rahami, Z.; Ghasemian, F.; Namazi, S.S.; Paknahad, A.; *et al.* Evaluation of attention-deficit hyperactivity disorder risk factors. *Int. J. Pediatr.* 2013, *2013*, 953103.
6. Scassellati, C.; Bonvicini, C.; Faraone, S.V.; Gennarelli, M. Biomarkers and attention-deficit/ hyperactivity disorder: A systematic review and meta-analyses. *J. Am. Acad. Child Adolesc. Psychiatry* 2012, *51*, 1003–1019.
7. Bradstreet, J.J.; Smith, S.; Baral, M.; Rossignol, D.A. Biomarker-guided interventions of clinically relevant conditions associated with autism spectrum disorders and attention deficit hyperactivity disorder. *Altern. Med. Rev.* 2010, *15*, 15–32.

8. Shaw, P.; Eckstrand, K.; Sharp, W.; Blumenthal, J.; Lerch, J.P.; Greenstein, D.; Clasen, L.; Evans, A.; Giedd, J.; Rapoport, J.L. Attention-deficit/hyperactivity disorder is characterized by a delay in cortical maturation. *Proc. Natl. Acad. Sci. USA* **2007**, *104*, 19649–19654.

9. Dickstein, S.G.; Bannon, K.; Castellanos, F.X.; Milham, M.P. The neural correlates of attention deficit hyperactivity disorder: An ALE meta-analysis. *J. Child Psychol. Psychiatry.* **2006**, *47*, 1051–1062.

10. Biederman, J.; Petty, C.R.; Woodworth, K.Y.; Lomedico, A.; Hyder, L.L.; Faraone, S.V. Adult outcome of attention-deficit/hyperactivity disorder: A controlled 16-year follow-up study. *J. Chin. Psychiatry* **2012**, *73*, 941–950.

11. Gjervan, B.; Torgersen, T.; Rasmussen, K.; Nordahl, H.M. Functional impairment and occupational outcome in adults with ADHD. *J. Atten. Discord.* **2012**, *16*, 544–552.

12. The MTA Cooperative Group. Moderators and mediators of treatment response for children with attention-deficit/hyperactivity disorder: The Multimodal Treatment study of children with Attention-deficit/hyperactivity disorder. *Arch. Gen. Psychiatry* **1999**, *56*, 1088–1096.

13. Sibley, M.H.; Kuriyan, A.B.; Evans, S.W.; Waxmonsky, J.G.; Smith, B.H. Pharmacological and psychosocial treatments for adolescents with ADHD: An updated systematic review of the literature. *Clin. Psychol. Rev.* **2014**, *34*, 218–232.

14. dosReis, S.; Owens, P.L.; Puccia, K.B.; Leaf, P.J. Multimodal treatment for ADHD among youths in three Medicaid subgroups: Disabled, foster care, and low income. *Psychiatr. Serv.* **2004**, *55*, 1041–1048.

15. Childress, A.C.; Sallee, F.R. Attention-deficit/hyperactivity disorder with inadequate response to stimulants: Approaches to management. **2014**, *28*, 121–129.

16. Toomey, S.L.; Sox, C.M.; Rusinak, D.; Finkelstein, J.A. Why do children with ADHD discontinue their medication? *Clin. Pediatr. (Phila.)* **2012**, *51*, 763–769.

17. National Institutes of Health: National Center for Complementary and Alternative Medicine (NCCAM) Children and Complementary Health Approaches. Available online: http://nccam.nih.gov/health/children (accessed on 17 March, 2014).

18. Chan, E.; Rappaport, L.A.; Kemper, K.J. Complementary and alternative therapies in childhood attention and hyperactivity problems. *J. Dev. Behav. Pediatr.* **2003**, *24*, 4–8.

19. Consortium of Academic Health Centers for Integrative medicine. Definition of Integrative Medicine. Available online: http://www.imconsortium.org/about/home.html (accessed on 17 March, 2014).

20. Millichap, J.G.; Yee, M.M. The diet factor in attention-deficit/hyperactivity disorder. *Pediatrics* **2012**, *129*, 330–337.

21. Cormier, E.; Elder, J.H. Diet and child behavior problems: Fact or fiction? *Pediatr. Nurs.* **2007**, *33*, 138–43.

22. Woo, H.D.; Kim, D.W.; Hong, Y.-S.; Kim, Y.-M.; Seo, J.-H.; Choe, B.M.; Park, J.H.; Kang, J.-W.; Yoo, J.-H.; Chueh, H.W.; *et al.* Dietary patterns in children with attention deficit/hyperactivity disorder (ADHD). *Nutrients* **2014**, *6*, 1539–1553.

23. Nigg, J.T.; Lewis, K.; Edinger, T.; Falk, M. Meta-analysis of attention-deficit/hyperactivity disorder or attention-deficit/hyperactivity disorder symptoms, restriction diet, and synthetic food color additives. *J. Am. Acad. Child Adolesc. Psychiatry* **2012**, *51*, 86–97.e8.

24. Schab, D.W.; Trinh, N.H. Do artificial food colors promote hyperactivity in children with hyperactive syndromes? A meta-analysis of double-blind placebo-controlled trials. *J. Dev. Behav. Pediatr.* **2004**, *25*, 423–434.

25. Arnold, L.E.; Hurt, E.; Lofthouse, N. Attention-deficit/hyperactivity disorder: Dietary and nutritional treatments. *Child Adolesc. Psychiatr. Clin. N. Am.* **2013**, *22*, 381–402.

26. Pelsser, L.M.; Frankena, K.; Toorman, J.; Savelkoul, H.F.; Dubois, A.E.; Pereira, R.R.; Haagen, T.A.; Rommelse, N.N.; Buitelaar, J.K. Effects of a restricted elimination diet on the behaviour of children with attention-deficit hyperactivity disorder (INCA study): A randomised controlled trial. *Lancet* **2011**, *377*, 494–503.

27. Howard, A.L.; Robinson, M.; Smith, G.J.; Ambrosini, G.L.; Piek, J.P.; Oddy, W.H. ADHD is associated with a "Western" dietary pattern in adolescents. *J. Atten. Disord.* **2011**, *15*, 403–411.

28. Melchior, M.; Chastang, J.F.; Falissard, B.; Galera, C.; Tremblay, R.E.; Cote, S.M.; Biovin, M. Food insecurity and children's mental health: A prospective cohort study. *PLoS One* **2012**, *7*, e52615.

29. Jacobson, M.F.; Schardt, D. *Diet, ADHD, & Behavior*; Center for Science in the Public Interest: Washington, DC, USA, 1999.

30. Verlaet, A.A.J.; Noriega, D.B.; Hermans, N.; Savelkoul, H.F.J. Nutrition, immunological mechanisms and dietary immunomodulation in ADHD. *Eur. Child Adolesc. Psychiatry* **2014**, *23*, 519–529.

31. Manzel, A.; Muller, D.N.; Hafler, D.A.; Erdman, S.E.; Linker, R.A.; Kleinewietfeld, M. Role of "Western diet" in inflammatory autoimmune diseases. *Curr. Allergy Asthma Rep.* **2014**, *14*, 404.

32. Mullin, G.E.; Swift, K.M.; Lipski, L.; Turnbull, L.K.; Rampertab, S.D. Testing for food reactions: The good, the bad, and the ugly. *Nutr. Clin. Pract.* **2010**, *25*, 192–198.

33. Sanford, N. *ADHD without Drugs: A Guide to the Natural Care of Children with ADHD*; Nurtured Heart Publications, Tucson, AZ, 2010.

34. Khalife, N.; Kantomaa, M.; Glover, V.; Tammelin, T.; Laitinen, J.; Ebeling, H.; Hurtig, T.; Jarvelin, M.R.; Rodriguez, A. Childhood attention-deficit/hyperactivity disorder symptoms are risk factors for obesity and physical inactivity in adolescence. *J. Am. Acad. Child Adolesc. Psychiatry* **2014**, *53*, 425–436.

35. Lobstein, T.; Dibb, S. Evidence of a possible link between obesogenic food advertising and child overweight. *Obes. Rev.* **2005**, *6*, 203–208.

36. Wiles, N.J.; Northstone, K.; Emmett, P.; Lewis, G.; Europe PMC Funders Group. "Junk food" diet and childhood behavioural problems: Results from the ALSPAC cohort. *Eur. J. Clin. Nutr.* **2009**, *63*, 491–498.

37. Conners, C.K.; Blouin, A.G. Nutritional effects on behavior of children. *J. Psychiatr. Res.* **1982–1983**, *17*, 193–201.

38. Wender, E.H.; Solanto, M.V. Effects of sugar on aggressive and inattentive behavior in children with attention deficit disorder with hyperactivity and normal children. *Pediatrics* **1991**, *88*, 960–966.

39. Wolraich, M.L.; Wilson, D.B.; White, J.W. The effect of sugar on behavior or cognition in children. A meta-analysis. *JAMA* **1995**, *4*, 1617–1621.

40. Lindseth, G.N.; Coolahan, S.E.; Petros, T.V.; Lindseth, P.D. Neurobehavioral Effects of Aspartame Consumption. *Res. Nurs. Health* **2014**, *37*, 185–193.

41. Humphries, P.; Pretorius, E.; Naudé, H. Direct and indirect cellular effects of aspartame on the brain. *Eur. J. Clin. Nutr.* **2008**, *62*, 451–462.

42. Kalaydjian, A.E.; Eaton, W.; Cascella, N.; Fasano, A. The gluten connection: The association between schizophrenia and celiac disease. *Acta Psychiatr. Scand.* **2006**, *113*, 82–90.

43. Jackson, J.R.; Eaton, W.W.; Cascella, N.G.; Fasano, A.; Kelly, D.L. Neurologic and psychiatric manifestations of celiac disease and gluten sensitivity. *Psychiatr. Q.* **2012**, *83*, 91–102.

44. Lachance, L.R.; McKenzie, K. Biomarkers of gluten sensitivity in patients with non-affective psychosis: A meta-analysis. *Schizophr. Res.* **2014**, *152*, 521–527.

45. Marí-Bauset, S.; Zazpe, I.; Mari-Sanchis, A.; Llopis-González, A.; Morales-Suárez-Varela, M. Evidence of the Gluten-Free and Casein-Free Diet in Autism Spectrum Disorders: A Systematic Review. *J. Child Neurol.* **2014**, doi: 10.1177/0883073814531330.

46. Rubio-Tapa, A.; Ludvigsson, J.; Brantner, T.; Murray, J.A.; Everhart, J.E. The prevalence of celiac disease in the United States. *Am. J. Gastroenterol.* **2012**, *107*, 1538–1544.

47. Tanpowpong, P.; Broder-Fingert, S.; Katz, A.J.; Camargo, C.A. Predictors of gluten avoidance and implementation of a gluten-free diet in children and adolescents without confirmed celiac disease. *J. Pediatr.* **2012**, *161*, 471–475.

48. Niederhofer, H. Association of attention-deficit/hyperactivity disorder and celiac disease: A brief report. *Prim. Care Companion CNS Disord.* **2011**, *13*, doi:10.4088/PCC.10br01104.

49. Niederhofer, H.; Pittschieler, K. A preliminary investigation of ADHD symptoms in persons with celiac disease. *J. Atten. Disord.* **2006**, *10*, 200–204.

50. Terrone, G.; Parente, I.; Romano, A.; Auricchio, R.; Greco, L.; del Giudice, E. The Pediatric Symptom Checklist as screening tool for neurological and psychosocial problems in a paediatric cohort of patients with coeliac disease. *Acta Paediatr.* **2013**, *102*, e325–e328.

51. Güngör, S.; Celiloğlu, O.S.; Ozcan, O.O.; Raif, S.G.; Selimoğlu, M.A. Frequency of celiac disease in attention-deficit/hyperactivity disorder. *J. Pediatr. Gastroenterol. Nutr.* **2013**, *56*, 211–214.

52. Carr, A.C. Depressed mood associated with gluten sensitivity—Resolution of symptoms with a gluten-free diet. *N. Z. Med. J.* **2012**, *125*, 81–82.

53. Pennesi, C.M.; Klein, L.C. Effectiveness of the gluten-free, casein-free diet for children diagnosed with autism spectrum disorder: Based on parental report. *Nutr. Neurosci.* **2012**, *15*, 85–91.

54. Genuis, S.J.; Lobo, R.A. Gluten Sensitivity Presenting as a Neuropsychiatric Disorder. *Gastroenterol. Res. Pract.* **2014**, *2014*, 293206:1–293206:6.

55. Rosen, A.; Sandstrom, O.; Carlsson, A.; Hogberg, L.; Olen, O.; Stenlund, H.; Ivarsson, A. Usefulness of Symptoms to Screen for Celiac Disease. *Pediatrics* **2014**, doi:10.1542/peds.2012-3765.

56. Ludvigsson, J.F.; Leffler, D.A.; Bai, J.; Biagi, F.; Fasano, A.; Green, P.H.; Hadjivassiliou, M.; Kaukinen, K.; Kelly, C.; Leonard, J.N.; *et al.* The Oslo definitions for coeliac disease and related terms. *Gut* **2013**, *62*, 43–52.

57. Sapone, A.; Bai, J.C.; Ciacci, C.; Dolinsek, J.; Green, P.H.R.; Hadjivassiliou, M.; Kaukinen, K.; Rostami, K.; Sanders, D.S.; Schumann, M.; *et al.* Spectrum of gluten-related disorders: Consensus on new nomenclature and classification. *BMC Med.* **2012**, *10*, 13.

58. Samsel, A.; Seneff, S. Glyphosate, pathways to modern diseases II: Celiac sprue and gluten intolerance. *Interdiscip. Toxicol.* **2013**, *6*, 159–184.

59. Mansueto, P.; Seidita, A. Non-Celiac Gluten Sensitivity: Literature Review. *J. Am. Coll. Nutr.* **2014**, *33*, 39–54.

60. Kurpad, A.V.; Edward, B.S.; Aeberli, I. Micronutrient supply and health outcomes in children. *Curr. Opin. Clin. Nutr. Metab. Care* **2013**, *16*, 328–338.

61. Anjos, T.; Altmäe, S.; Emmett, P.; Tiemeier, H.; Closa-Monasterolo, R.; Luque, V.; Wiseman, S.; Pérez-García, M.; Lattka, E.; Demmelmair, H.; *et al.* Nutrition and neurodevelopment in children: Focus on NUTRIMENTHE project. *Eur. J. Nutr.* **2013**, *52*, 1825–1842.

62. Lord, R.S.; Brailey, J.A. *Laboratory Evaluations for Integrative and Functional Medicine*, 2nd ed.; Metametrix Institute, Duluth, GA, 2008.

63. Thomas, D. The mineral depletion of foods available to us as a nation (1940–2002)—A review of the 6th Edition of McCance and Widdowson. *Nutr. Health* **2007**, *19*, 21–55.

64. Corbo, M.D.; Lam, J. Zinc deficiency and its management in the pediatric population: A literature review and proposed etiologic classification. *J. Am. Acad. Dermatol.* **2013**, *69*, 616–624.e1.

65. Lepping, P.; Huber, M. Role of zinc in the pathogenesis of attention-deficit hyperactivity disorder. *CNS Drugs* **2010**, *24*, 721–728.

66. Bitanihirwe, B.K.Y.; Cunningham, M.G. Zinc: The brain's dark horse. *Synapse* **2009**, *63*, 1029–1049.

67. Wessells, K.R.; Singh, G.M.; Brown, K.H. Estimating the global prevalence of inadequate zinc intake from national food balance sheets: Effects of methodological assumptions. *PLoS One* **2012**, *7*, e50565.

68. Mahmoud, M.M.; el-Mazary, A.-A.M.; Maher, R.M.; Saber, M.M. Zinc, ferritin, magnesium and copper in a group of Egyptian children with attention deficit hyperactivity disorder. *Ital. J. Pediatr.* **2011**, *37*, 60.

69. Sarris, J.; Kean, J.; Schweitzer, I.; Lake, J. Complementary medicines (herbal and nutritional products) in the treatment of Attention Deficit Hyperactivity Disorder (ADHD): A systematic review of the evidence. *Complement. Ther. Med.* **2011**, *19*, 216–227.

70. Searight, H.R.; Robertson, K.; Smith, T.; Perkins, S.; Searight, B.K. Complementary and alternative therapies for pediatric attention deficit hyperactivity disorder: A descriptive review. *ISRN Psychiatry* **2012**, *2012*, 804127.

71. Gogia, S.; Sachdev, H.S. Zinc supplementation for mental and motor development in children. *Cochrane Database Syst. Rev.* **2012**, *12*, CD007991.

72. Bilici, M.; Yildrim, F.; Kandil, S.; Bekaroglu, M.; Yildirmis, S.; Deger, O.; Ulgen, M.; Yildiran, A.; Aksu, H. Double-blind, placebo-controlled study of zinc sulfate in the treatment of attention deficit hyperactivity disorder. *Prog. Neuropsychopharmacol. Biol. Psychiatry* **2004**, *28*, 181–190.

73. Akhondzadeh, S.; Mohammadi, M.R.; Khademi, M. Zinc sulfate as an adjunct to methylphenidate for the treatment of attention deficit hyperactivity disorder in children: A double blind and randomized trial. *BMC Psychiatry* **2004**, *4*, 90.

74. Arnold, L.E.; Disilvestro, R.A.; Bozzolo, D.; Bozzolo, H.; Crowl, L.; Fernandez, S.; Ramadan, Y.; Thompson, S.; Mo, X.; Abdel-Rasoul, M.; *et al.* Zinc for attention-deficit/hyperactivity disorder: Placebo-controlled double-blind pilot trial alone and combined with amphetamine. *J. Child Adolesc. Psychopharmacol.* **2011**, *21*, 1–19.

75. Youdim, M.B. Iron deficiency effects on brain function. *Public Health Rev.* **2000**, *28*, 83–88.

76. Calarge, C.; Farmer, C.; DiSilvestro, R.; Arnold, L.E. Serum ferritin and amphetamien response in youth with attention-deficit/hyperactivity disorder. *J. Child Adolesc. Psychopharmacol.* **2010**, *20*, 495–502.

77. Cortese, S.; Konofal, E.; Bernardina, B.D.; Mouren, M.C.; Lecendreux, M. Sleep disturbances and serum ferritin levels in children with attention-deficit/hyperactivity disorder. *Eur. Child Adolesc. Psychiatry* **2009**, *18*, 393–399.

78. Hentze, M.W.; Muckenthaler, M.U.; Galy, B.; Camaschella, C. Two to tango: Regulation of Mammalian iron metabolism. *Cell* **2010**, *142*, 24–38.

79. Dolina, S.; Margalit, D.; Malitsky, S.; Rabinkov, A. Attention-deficit hyperactivity disorder (ADHD) as a pyridoxine-dependent condition: Urinary diagnostic biomarkers. *Med. Hypotheses* **2014**, *82*, 111–116.

80. Manor, L.; Newcorn, J.H.; Faraone, S.V.; Adler, L.A. Efficacy of metadoxine extended release in patients with predominantly inattentive subtype attention-deficit/hyperactivity disorder. *Postgrad. Med.* **2013**, *125*, 181–190.

81. Volpe, S.L. Magnesium in disease prevention and overall health. *Adv. Nutr.* **2013**, *1*, 378s–383s.

82. Starobrat-Hermelin, B.; Kozielec, T. The effects of magnesium physiological supplementation on hyperactivity in children with ADHD: Positive response to magnesium oral loading test. *Magnes. Res.* **1997**, *10*, 149–156.

83. Mousain-Bosc, M.; Roche, M.; Rapin, J.; Bali, J.P. Magnesium VitB6 intake reduces central nervous system hyperexcitability in children. *J. Am. Coll. Nutr.* **2004**, *23*, 545S–548S.

84. Nogovitsina, O.R.; Levitina, E.V. Neurological aspects of the clinical features, pathophysiology, and corrections of impairments in attention deficit hyperactivity disorder. *Neurosci. Behav. Physiol.* **2007**, *37*, 199–202.

85. Clerc, P.; Young, C.A.; Bordt, E.A.; Grigore, A.M.; Fiskum, G.; Polster, B.M. Magnesium sulfate protects against the bioenergetic consequences of chronic glutamate receptor stimulation. *PLoS One* **2013**, *8*, e79982.

86. Kozielec, T.; Starobrat-Hermelin, B. Assessment of magnesium levels in children with attention deficit hyperactivity disorder (ADHD). *Magnes. Res.* **1997**, *10*, 143–148.

87. Ghanizadeh, A. A Systematic Review of Magnesium Therapy for Treating Attention Deficit Hyperactivity Disorder. *Arch. Iran. Med.* **2013**, *16*, 412–417.

88. Galland, L. Diet and inflammation. *Nutr. Clin. Pract.* **2010**, *25*, 634–640.

89. Simopoulos, A.P. Evolutionary aspects of diet: The omega-6/omega-3 ratio and the brain. *Mol. Neurobiol.* **2011**, *44*, 203–215.

90. Kapoor, R.; Huang, Y.S. Gamma linolenic acid: An antinflammatory omega-6 fatty acid. *Curr. Pharm. Biotechnol.* **2006**, *7*, 531–534.

91. Stipanuk, M.H. *Biochemical, Physiological, & Molecular Aspects of Human Nutrition*, 2nd ed.; Saunders by Elsevier, Inc.: St. Louis, MO, USA, 2006.

92. Strobel, C.; Jahreis, G.; Kuhnt, K. Survey of n-3 and n-6 polyunsaturated fatty acids in fish and fish products. *Lipids Health Dis.* **2011**, *11*, 144.

93. Carlson, S.J.; Fallon, E.M.; Kalish, B.T.; Gura, K.M.; Puder, M. The role of the ω-3 fatty acid DHA in the human life cycle. *JPEN J. Parenter. Enteral Nutr.* **2013**, *37*, 15–22.

94. Mitchell, R.H.B.; Goldstein, B.I. Inflammation in Children and Adolescents with Neuropsychiatric Disorders: A Systematic Review. *J. Am. Acad. Child Adolesc. Psychiatry* **2014**, *53*, 274–296.

95. Bloch, M.H.; Qawasami, A. Omega-3 fatty acid supplementation for the treatment of children with attention-deficity/hyperactivity disorder symptomatology: Systematic review and meta-analysis. *J. Am. Acad. Child Adolesc. Psychiatry* **2011**, *50*, 991–1000.

96. Gustafsson, P.A.; Birberg-Thornberg, U.; Duchen, K.; Landgren, M.; Malmberg, K.; Pelling, H.; Strandvik, B.; Karlsson, T. EPA supplementation improves teacher-rated behavior and oppositional symptoms in children with ADHD. *Acta Paediatr.* **2010**, *99*, 1540–1549.

97. Milte, C.M.; Parletta, N.; Buckley, J.D.; Coates, A.M.; Young, R.M.; Howe, P.R. Eicosapentaenoic and docosahexaenoic acids, cognition, and behavior in children with attention-deficit/hyperactivity disorder: A randomized controlled trial. *Nutrition* **2012**, *28*, 670–677.

98. Widenhorn-Muller, K.; Schwanda, S.; Scholz, E.; Spitzer, M.; Bode, H. Effect of supplementation with long-chain ω-3 polyunsaturated fatty acids on behavior and cognition in children with attention deficit/hyperactivity disorder (ADHD): A randomized placebo-controlled intervention trial. *Prostaglandins Leukot. Essent. Fatty Acids* **2014**, *91*, 49–60.

99. Stevens, L.; Zhang, W.; Peck, L.; Kuczek, T.; Grevstad, N.; Mahon, A.; Zentall, S.S.; Arnold, L.E.; Burgess, J.R. EFA supplementation in children with inattention, hyperactivity and other disruptive behaviors. *Lipids* **2003**, *38*, 1007–1021.

100. Raz, R.; Carasso, R.L.; Yehuda, S. The influence of short-chain essential fatty acids on children with attention-deficit/hyperactivity disorder: A double-blind placebo-controlled study. *J. Child Adolesc. Psychopharmacol.* **2009**, *19*, 167–177.

101. Gillies, D.; Sinn, J.K.H.; Lad, S.S.; Leach, M.J.; Ross, M.J. Polyunsaturated fatty acids (PUFA) for attention deficit hyperactivity disorder (ADHD) in children and adolescents. *Cochrane Database Syst. Rev.* **2012**, *7*, CD007986.

102. Schachter, H.M.; Pham, B.; King, J.; Langford, S.; Moher, D. How efficacious and safe is short-acting methylphenidate for the treatment of attention-deficit disorder in children and adolescents? A meta-analysis. *CMAJ* **2001**, *164*, 1475–1488.
103. Vaisman, N.; Kaysar, N.; Zaruk-Adasha, Y.; Pelled, D.; Brichon, G.; Zwingelstein, G.; Bodennec, J. Correlation between changes in blood fatty acid composition and visual sustained attention performance in children with inattention: Effect of dietary n-3 fatty acids containing phospholipids. *Am. J. Clin. Nutr.* **2008**, *87*, 1170–1180.
104. Harris, W.S. Expert opinion: Omega-3 fatty acids and bleeding-cause for concern? *Am. J. Cardiol.* **2007**, *99*, 44C–46C.
105. Gorini, A.; D'Angelo, A.; Villa, R.F. Energy metabolism of synaptosomal subpopulations from different neuronal systems of rat hippocampus: Effect of L-acetylcarnitine administration *in vivo*. *Neurochem. Res.* **1999**, *24*, 617–624.
106. Juliet, P.A.; Balasubramaniam, D.; Balasubramaniam, N.; Panneerselvam, C. Carnitine: A neuromodulator in aged rats. *J. Gerontol. A Biol. Sci. Med. Sci.* **2003**, *58*, 970–974.
107. Arnold, L.E.; Amato, A.; Bozzolo, H.; Hollway, J.; Cook, A.; Ramadan, Y.; Crowl, L.; Zhang, D.; Thompson, S.; Testa, G.; *et al.* Acetyl-L-carnitine (ALC) in attention-deficit/hyperactivity disorder: A multi-site, placebo-controlled pilot trial. *J. Child Adolesc. Psychopharmacol.* **2007**, *17*, 791–802.
108. Van Oudheusden, L.J.; Scholte, H.R. Efficacy of carnitine in the treatment of children with attention-deficit hyperactivity disorder. **2002**, *67*, 33–38.
109. Abassi, S.H.; Heidari, S.; Mohammadi, M.R.; Tabrizi, M.; Ghaleiha, A.; Akhondzadeh, S. Acetyl-L-carnitine as an adjunctive therapy in the treatment of attention-deficit/hyperactivity disorder in children and adolescents: A placebo-controlled trial. *Child Psychiatry Hum. Dev.* **2011**, *42*, 367–375.
110. Kamal, M.; Bener, A.; Ehlayel, M.S. Is high prevalence of vitamin D deficiency a correlate for attention deficit hyperactivity disorder? *Atten. Defic. Hyperact. Disord.* **2014**, *6*, 73–78.
111. Hewison, M. Vitamin D and immune function: An overview. *Proc. Nutr. Soc.* **2012**, *71*, 50–61.
112. Eyles, D.W.; Feron, F.; Cui, X.; Kesby, J.P.; Harms, L.H.; Ko, P.; McGrath, J.J.; Burne, T.H.J. Developmental vitamin D deficiency causes abnormal brain development. *Psychoneuroendocrinology* **2009**, *34* (Suppl. 1), S247–S257.
113. Taylor, A.F.; Kuo, F.E. A potential natural treatment for attention-deficit/hyperactivity disorder: Evidence from a national study. *Am. J. Public Health* **2004**, *94*, 1580–1586.
114. Caldwell, K.L.; Makhmudov, A.; Ely, E.; Jones, R.L.; Wang, R.Y. Iodine status of the U.S. population, National Health and Nutrition Examination Survey, 2005–2006 and 2007–2008. *Thyroid* **2011**, *21*, 419–427.
115. Verheesen, R.H.; Schweitzer, C.M. Iodine deficiency, more than cretinism and goiter. *Med. Hypotheses* **2008**, *71*, 645–648.
116. Walsh, C.J.; Guinane, C.M.; O'Toole, P.W.; Cotter, P.D. Beneficial modulation of the gut microbiota. *FEBS Lett.* **2014**, doi:10.1016/j.febslet.2014.03.035.

117. Tillisch, K.; Labus, J.; Kilpatrick, L.; Jiang, Z.; Stains, J.; Ebrat, B.; Guonnet, D.; Legrain-Raspaud, S.; Trotin, B.; Naliboff, B.; *et al.* Consumption of fermented milk product with probiotic modulates brain activity. **2013**, *144*, 1394–1401.

118. Gonzalez, A.; Stombaugh, J.; Lozupone, C.; Turnbaugh, P.J.; Gordon, J.I.; Knight, R. The mind-body-microbial continuum. *Dialogues Clin. Neurosc.* **2011**, *13*, 55–62.

119. Lyte, M. Probiotics function mechanistically as delivery vehicles for neuroactive compounds: Microbial endocrinology in the design and use of probiotics. *Bioessays* **2011**, *33*, 574–581.

120. Farmer, A.D.; Randall, H.A.; Aziz, Q. It's a Gut Feeling—How the gut microbiota affects the state of mind SHORT TITLE. *J. Physiol.* **2014**, *592*, 2981-2988.

121. Biasucci, G.; Rubini, M.; Riboni, S.; Morelli, L.; Bessi, E.; Retetangos, C. Mode of delivery affects the bacterial community in the newborn gut. *Early Hum. Dev.* **2010**, *86* (Suppl. 1), 13–15.

122. Amiri, S.; Malek, A.; Sadegfard, M.; Abdi, S. Pregnancy-related maternal risk factors of attention-deficit hyperactivity disorder: A case-control study. *ISRN Pediatr.* **2012**, *2012*, 458064.

123. Berick, P.; Collins, S.M. Microbial Endocrinology: The microbiota-gut-brain axis in health and disease. *Adv. Exp. Med. Biol.* **2014**, *817*, 279–289.

124. Rucklidge, J.J. Could yeast infections impair recovery from mental illness? A case study using micronutrients and olive leaf extract for the treatment of ADHD and depression. *Adv. Mind Body Med.* **2013**, *27*, 14–18.

125. David, L.A.; Maurice, C.F.; Carmody, R.N.; Gootenberg, D.B.; Button, J.E.; Wolfe, B.E.; Ling, A.V.; Devlin, A.S.; Varma, Y.; Fischbach, M.A.; *et al.* Diet rapidly and reproducibly alters the human gut microbiome. *Nature* **2013**, *505*, 559–563.

126. DATA.GOV. "Toxic Substances Control Act (TSCA) Inventory". Available online: https://explore.data.gov/Geography-and-Environment/TSCA-Inventory/pkhi-wvjh (accessed on 12 May, 2014).

127. Centers for Disease Control and Prevention, Department of Health and Human Services (2009). "Fourth National Report on Human Exposure to Environmental Chemicals". Available online: http://www.cdc.gov/exposurereport/pdf/fourthreport.pdf (accessed on 12 May, 2014).

128. Grandjean, P.; Landrigan, P.J. Developmental neurotoxicity of industrial chemicals. *Lancet* **2006**, *368*, 2167–2178.

129. Gilbert, S.G.; Miller, E.; Martin, J.; Abulafia, L. Scientific and policy statements on environmental agents associated with neurodevelopmental disorders. *J. Intellect. Dev. Disabil.* **2010**, *35*, 121–128.

130. Sagiv, S.K.; Thurston, S.W.; Bellinger, D.C.; Tolbert, P.E.; Altshul, L.M.; Korrick, S.A. Prenatal organochlorine exposure and behaviors associated with attention deficit hyperactivity disorder in school-aged children. *Am. J. Epidemiol.* **2010**, *171*, 593–601.

131. Aguiar, A.; Eubig, P.A.; Schantz, S.L. Attention deficit/hyperactivity disorder: A focused overview for children's environmental health researchers. *Environ. Health Perspect.* **2010**, *118*, 1646–1653.

132. Bouchard, M.F.; Bellinger, D.C.; Wright, R.O.; Weisskopf, M.G. Attention-deficit/hyperactivity disorder and urinary metabolites of organophosphate pesticides. *Pediatrics* **2010**, *125*, e1270–e1277.

133. Lu, C.; Toepel, K.; Irish, R.; Fenske, R.A.; Barr, D.B.; Bravo, R. Organic Diets Significantly Lower Children's Dietary Exposure to Organophosphorus Pesticides. *Environ. Health Perspect.* **2006**, *114*, 260–263.

134. United States Department of Agriculture. 2014. *Pesticide Data Program: Annual Summary, Calendar Year 2012*; U.S. Department of Agriculture: Washington, DC, USA, 2014.

135. Environmental Working Group. Executive Summary: EWG's 2014 Shopper's Guide to Pesticides in Produce. Available online: http://www.eg.org/foodnews/summary.php (accessed on 14 April, 2014).

136. De Cock, M.; Maas, Y.G.H.; van de Bor, M. Does perinatal exposure to endocrine disruptors induce autism spectrum and attention deficit hyperactivity disorders? Review. *Acta Paediatr.* **2012**, *101*, 811–818.

137. Niggs, J.T. Childhood blood lead levels. *J. Child Psychol. Psychiatry* **2010**, *51*, 58–65.

138. Schnur, J.; John, R.M. Childhood lead poisoning and the new Centers for Disease Control and Prevention guidelines for lead exposure. *J. Am. Assoc. Nurse Pract.* **2014**, *26*, 238–247.

139. Lofthouse, N.; Arnold, L.E.; Hersch, S.; Hurt, E.; DeBeus, R. A review of neurofeedback treatment for pediatric ADHD. *J. Atten. Disord.* **2012**, *16*, 351–372.

140. Kim, B.N.; Lee, J.S.; Shin, M.S.; Cho, S.C.; Lee, D.S. Regional cerebral perfusion abnormalities in attention deficit/hyperactivity disorder. Statistical parametric mapping analysis. *Eur. Arch. Psychiatry Clin. Neurosci.* **2002**, *252*, 219–225.

141. Lubar, J.F.; Shouse, M.N. EEG and behavioral changes in a hyperkinetic child concurrent with training of the senorimotor rhythm (SMR): A preliminary report. *Biofeedback Self Regul.* **1976**, *1*, 293–306.

142. U.S. Food and Drug Administration (2013): FDA Permits Marketing of First Brain Wave Test to Help Assess Children and Teens for ADHD. Available online: http://www.fda.gov/newsevents/newsroom/pressannouncements/ucm360811.htm (accessed on 12 May, 2014).

143. Loo, S.K.; Makeig, S. Clinical utility of EEG in attention-deficit/hyperactivity disorder: A research update. *Neurotherapeutics* **2012**, *9*, 569–587.

144. Ogrim, G.; Hestad, K.A. Effects of Neurofeedback *versus* Stimulant Medication in Attention-Deficit/Hyperactivity Disorder: A Randomized Pilot Study. *J. Child Adolesc. Psychopharmacol.* **2013**, *27*, 448–457.

145. Arns, M.; Conners, C.K.; Kraemer, H.C. A decade of EEG Theta/Beta Ratio Research in ADHD: A meta-analysis. *J. Atten. Disord.* **2013**, *17*, 374–383.

146. Loo, S.K.; Barkley, R.A. Clinical utility of EEG in attention deficit hyperactivity disorder. *Appl. Neuropsychol.* **2005**, *12*, 64–76.

147. Ogrim, G.; Kropotov, J.; Brunner, J.F.; Candrian, G.; Sandvik, L.; Hestad, K.A. Predicting the clinical outcome of stimulant medication in pediatric attention-deficit/hyperactivity disorder: Data from quantitative electroencephalography, event-related potentials, and a go/no-go test. *Neuropsychiatr. Dis. Treat.* **2014**, *10*, 231–242.

148. Heinrich, H.; Gevensleben, H.; Freisleder, F.J.; Moll, G.H.; Rothenberger, A. Training of slow cortical potentials in attention-deficit/hyperactivity disorder: Evidence for positive behavioral and neurophysiological effects. *Biol. Psychiatry* **2004**, *55*, 772–775.

149. Birbaumer, N.; Elbert, T.; Canavan, A.; Rockstroh, B. Slow potentials of the cerebral cortex and behavior. *Physiol. Rev.* **1990**, *70*, 1–41.

150. Gevensleben, H.; Holl, B.; Albrecht, B.; Vogel, C.; Schlamp, D.; Kratz, O.; Studer, P.; Rothenberger, A.; Moll, G.H.; Heinrich, H. Is neurofeedback an efficacious treatment for ADHD? A randomised controlled clinical trial. *J. Child Psychol. Psychiatry* **2009**, *50*, 780–789.

151. Mayer, K.; Wyckoff, S.N.; Strehl, U. One size fits all? Slow cortical potentials neurofeedback: A review. *J. Atten. Disord.* **2013**, *17*, 393–409.

152. Meisel, V.; Servera, M.; Garcia-Banda, G.; Cardo, E.; Moreno, I. Neurofeedback and standard pharmacological intervention in ADHD: A randomized controlled trial with six-month follow-up. *Biol. Psychol.* **2013**, *94*, 12–21.

153. Gevensleben, H.; Kleemeyer, M.; Rothenberger, L.G.; Studer, P.; Flaig-Röhr, A.; Moll, G.H.; Rothenberger, A.; Heinrich, H. Neurofeedback in ADHD: Further Pieces of the Puzzle. *Brain Topogr.* **2014**, *27*, 20–32.

154. Patsopoulos, N.A. A pragmatic view on pragmatic trials. *Dialogues Clin Neurosci* **2011**, *13*, 217–224.

155. Heaney, R.P. Guidelines for optimizing design and analysis of clinical studies of nutrient effects. *Nutr. Rev.* **2014**, *72*, 48–54.

Integrative Therapies and Pediatric Inflammatory Bowel Disease: The Current Evidence

Sanghamitra M. Misra

Abstract: Inflammatory bowel disease (IBD) primarily describes two distinct chronic conditions with unknown etiology, ulcerative colitis (UC) and Crohn's disease (CD). UC is limited to the colon, while CD may involve any portion of the gastrointestinal tract from mouth to anus. These diseases exhibit a pattern of relapse and remission, and the disease processes are often painful and debilitating. Due to the chronic nature of IBD and the negative side effects of many of the conventional therapies, many patients and their families turn to complementary and alternative medicine (CAM) for symptom relief. This article focuses on the current available evidence behind CAM/integrative therapies for IBD.

Reprinted from *Children*. Cite as: Misra, S.M. Integrative Therapies and Pediatric Inflammatory Bowel Disease: The Current Evidence. *Children* **2014**, *1*, 149-165.

1. Introduction

Inflammatory bowel disease (IBD) primarily describes two distinct chronic conditions with unknown etiology, ulcerative colitis (UC) and Crohn's disease (CD). UC is limited to the colon, while CD may involve any portion of the gastrointestinal tract from mouth to anus. These diseases exhibit a pattern of relapse and remission, and the disease processes are often painful and debilitating. The peak incidence of IBD is in patients between the ages of 15 and 25 years. Approximately 25% to 30% of patients with CD and 20% of patients with UC present before the age of 20 years [1]. Unfortunately, children with IBD are generally more likely than adults to present with extensive intestinal involvement and have rapid clinical progression [2,3].

The pathogenesis of CD and UC are not well understood; however, a combination of genetics and environmental factors likely play a role in development of IBD. Genetic predisposition to IBD has been studied extensively. Multiple population studies have shown that relatives of patients with IBD have a significantly higher risk of developing the same condition when compared to the general population [4–6]. According to Nunes *et al.* "familial aggregation has been more frequently reported in CD than UC. In first degree relatives, the age-adjusted relative risk of developing the same type of IBD ranges from 2 to 8 for UC and from 5 to 10 in the case of CD [7–10]". Twin studies have effectively demonstrated the genetic influence on the development of IBD. In a Swedish twin cohort study of 80 twins with IBD, the concordance rate for monozygotic twins was markedly higher in CD than UC (50% *versus* 19%) and continued to rise over time [11]. The greatest IBD concordance rates have been shown among monozygotic twins, ranging from 20% to 50% in CD and from 14% to 19% in UC twins, whereas in dizygotic twins, concordance rates are as low as 0%–7% in CD and UC twins [12,13]. In an analysis of populations, the prevalence of IBD among the Jewish population is 2 to 4 times higher than in any other ethnic group, being greater in the Ashkenazi than in any other Jewish group [4,9].

Numerous theories are emerging on possible environmental factors in the development of IBD, including the use of NSAIDs, the hygiene hypothesis, and early exposure to antibiotics. Although it has not been studied extensively in children, the use of NSAIDs may play a role in the development of IBD. From the prospective cohort study, Nurses' Health Study I, with data from more than 75,000 women, frequent use of NSAIDs, but not aspirin, seemed to be associated with increased absolute incidence of CD and UC [14]. In those with IBD, NSAIDs have been shown to exacerbate UC and CD symptoms [15]. However, one study in adults concluded that psychological factors contribute to IBD symptom flares and that there was no support for differential rates of the use of NSAIDS, antibiotics or for the occurrence of non-enteric infections related to IBD flares [16]. The hygiene hypothesis proposes that the increasing frequency of immunologic disorders can be attributed to decreased childhood exposure to pathogens and, particularly, enteric pathogens. A few studies have shown that exposure to farm animals early in life may be protective against IBD [17,18]. One study showed a strong protective effect of worm infestations for the occurrence of CD, but not UC [19]. A 2006 study showed that having pet cats before the age of five may be protective against CD [20]. There is emerging concern that early antibiotic use may also alter the immune system and result in autoimmune diseases and IBD. A study by Shaw et al. showed that of 36 children with IBD, 21 children (58%) had one or more antibiotic dispensations in their first year of life compared with 39% of controls. Crohn's disease was diagnosed in 75% of the IBD cases, and those receiving one or more dispensations of antibiotics were at 2.9-times the odds of being an IBD case [21]. The development of IBD is multifactorial, andcontinuing research is needed to better understand the pathophysiology of CD and UC. A more complete understanding of the development of IBD may help create more effective treatments for IBD.

2. Conventional Treatment

Allopathic treatment of IBD generally includes corticosteroids to induce remission and 5-aminosalicylic acid (5-ASA) agents, also known as mesalamines, as maintenance therapy. Alternative agents, such as 6-mercaptopurine and azathioprine, are used in more severe disease unresponsive to 5-ASA agents. In patients unresponsive to the above therapies, anti-tumor necrosis factor (TNF) monoclonal antibodies can be effective, but these drugs carry risk of malignancies and severe infections due to their effects on the immune system. Due to the chronic nature of IBD and the negative side effects of many of the conventional therapies, many patients and their families turn to complementary and alternative medicine (CAM) for symptom relief. The incidence of CAM use in pediatric IBD patients from a 2009 multicenter study was 50% [22]. Previous studies documented CAM use in pediatric IBD ranging from 40% to 72% [23,24]. A 2014 survey study of adolescent patients with IBD showed that during the preceding 12 months, 48% regularly used CAM, while 81% reported occasional CAM use [25]. Practitioners caring for pediatric IBD patients should be aware that their patients may be using alternative therapies.

3. Integrative Treatment

The integrative treatment of IBD is highly individualized and addresses the "whole" person with a focus on improving quality of life. Integrative practitioners consider a wide array of factors when prescribing a course of treatment. Thorough evaluation of the underlying disorder is the initial step to creating a treatment plan. Assessment of the patient's diet includes food intolerances and gut permeability, as well as consideration for optimal nutrition and potential nutritional deficiencies. Stool studies, which evaluate the gut flora, specifically the overgrowth of bacteria, are also vital in guiding treatment. Often, understanding which symptoms are most bothersome to the patient helps focus the treatment plan. Herbs and supplements are prescribed if expected to be beneficial and generally considered to be safe. As the field of integrative pediatrics is newly emerging, there are few large studies investigating the safety and efficacy of certain herbs or therapies for particular disease processes. Therefore, practitioners often balance risk and benefit and offer a trial of an herb or therapy that may benefit a patient. In the integrative model, all available interventions are utilized to create a successful plan of care with emphasis on empowering the patient. This article will focus on the current available evidence behind CAM/integrative therapies for IBD.

4. Breastfeeding

Many researchers have investigated the relationship of IBD with breastfeeding exposure. Early studies suggested that IBD patients were less likely to have been breastfed as infants. Koletzko *et al.* found that children with CD were more than three times less likely to have been breastfed than their unaffected siblings [26]; however, no association was found between breastfeeding history and the risk of developing UC in childhood [27]. A systematic review examining early-onset IBD (<16 years at diagnosis) concluded that breast milk may be protective, but the quality of existing data is generally poor [28].

5. Diet

Diet and nutrition are important aspects of IBD management. As IBD involves the GI tract, patients often search for diets that will alleviate their symptoms. There is no evidence that inflammation of the intestines is directly related to particular foods. However, certain foods may worsen symptoms due to food allergy or food intolerance. Many IBD patients follow a normal diet, but avoid those foods that tend to exacerbate their symptoms. These elimination diets can be helpful, but patients should be cautioned against diets that are so restrictive that they result in nutritional deficiencies. Many IBD patients learn from trial and error which foods they tolerate well and which foods result in GI distress. As food intolerances are usually inconsistent among IBD patients, general dietary recommendations cannot be made for all IBD patients.

Some patients with IBD avoid milk products, because they suffer from lactose intolerance or experience exacerbation of symptoms from milk products. Inadequate calcium intake is present in one-third of IBD patients [29]. Restricting milk products can have negative effects, as it may lead to calcium and vitamin D deficiency [30]. Lactase enzyme supplements can be recommended for better tolerance of milk products.

A common conventional diet option for IBD patients is the low-fiber with low-residue diet. This includes decreasing the intake of raw foods, like fruits, vegetables and nuts, that add bulk residue to stool. This diet may be helpful during flares and for patients with bowel strictures. Families often turn to other diets, like the Maker's diet, the Specific Carbohydrate Diet^{TM} and the Colitis Five-Step formula. The Maker's Diet, also known as the Bible diet, focuses on physical, mental, spiritual and emotional health. The diet recommendations include foods that are unprocessed, unrefined and untreated with pesticides or hormones. The Maker's Diet may be beneficial for patients, but its efficacy has not been studied in children with IBD. The Specific Carbohydrate Diet^{TM} (SCD) is "based on the principle that specifically selected carbohydrates, requiring minimal digestive processes, are well absorbed and leave virtually none to be used for furthering microbial overgrowth in the intestine. As the microbial population decreases due to lack of food, its harmful byproducts also decrease, freeing the intestinal surface of injurious substances. No longer needing protection, the mucus-producing cells stop producing excessive mucus, and carbohydrate digestion is improved. Malabsorption is replaced by absorption" [31]. Evidence shows that the SCD is more effective in CD than in UC. A chart review by Suskind et al. suggests that the SCD and other low complex carbohydrate diets may be possible therapeutic options for pediatric Crohn's disease [32]. A prospective pilot study of the SCD in children with Crohn's disease showed clinical and mucosal improvements in children with CD using the SCD over 12 and 52 weeks [33]. The Colitis Five-Step formula believes in the elimination of infection with a "natural pathogen killer." If used with proper diet and physical activity, the formula can put the digestive system back in order. This diet has not been studied in pediatric IBD. The use of any special diet in children with IBD should be coordinated with a knowledgeable practitioner.

Exclusive enteral nutrition (EEN) is the consumption of an elemental or polymeric formula, with the exclusion of all other nutrients, for a period of up to 12 weeks. EEN has become an established and reliable option for the treatment of pediatric IBD [34]. In CD, but not in UC, enteral feeding of defined formula diets as a primary therapy has been shown to induce the remission of active disease. There have been several randomized controlled trials comparing EEN to standard treatment. A study from the Netherlands of 77 Crohn's disease pediatric patients investigated EEN as either hyperosmolar sip feeds or polymeric formula by a nasogastric tube. In patients completing a six-week course of EEN ($n = 58$), complete remission was achieved in 71%, partial remission in 26% and no response was seen in 3%. The authors concluded that a six-week course of EEN is effective in newly diagnosed pediatric CD, with response rates that seem to be influenced by disease location and nutritional status, but not by type of formula [35]. A study by Knight et al. investigated the long-term benefits of EEN in 44 patients. Forty out of 44 patients (90%) responded to enteral nutrition, with a median time to remission of six weeks. Twenty five of these 40 (62%) relapsed, with a median duration of remission of 54.5 weeks (range 4–312). Fifteen (38%) had not relapsed. Twenty one of the 44 (47%) had not received steroids. In those who eventually required steroids, their use was postponed for a median 68 weeks (range 6–190). The authors concluded that EEN can postpone or prevent the need for steroids [36]. A review of five randomized clinical trials in 2000 concluded that "there is no difference in efficacy between enteral nutrition and corticosteroid therapy in the treatment of acute Crohn's disease in children. Improved growth and development, without the side effects of steroid therapy, make enteral nutrition a better choice for first-line therapy in children with active Crohn's disease" [37]. A meta-analysis in 2007 also concluded that limited data suggest similar efficacy for EN and corticosteroids [38].

Vitamin supplementation can be beneficial for IBD patients. In general, a daily multivitamin may help improve overall nutritional status. Folic acid deficiency is common in patients taking sulfasalazines. Therefore, all patients on sulfasalazine should take daily folic acid supplementation. Many IBD patients are deficient in vitamin D due to corticosteroid use, malabsorption or lack of sun exposure. IBD patients are also commonly deficient in calcium, sometimes due to avoidance of dairy products. Vitamin D and calcium supplementation are often necessary in children with IBD to ensure optimal growth and healing. Patients with CD and ileal inflammation are often deficient in Vitamin B12 and require supplementation.

6. Fish Oil (Polyunsaturated Fatty Acids)

Because of their anti-inflammatory action, omega-3 polyunsaturated fatty acids (PUFAs) may be beneficial in IBD. Of note, the incidence rates of IBD are lower in countries with high fish consumption, like Japan [39]. One study showed that children with IBD have a high risk of omega-6 PUFA depletion, which is related to disease activity [40]. A study by Uchiyama et al. in 2010 concluded that an n-3 PUFA food exchange table (N-3DP) significantly increased the erythrocyte membrane n-3/n-6 ratio in IBD patients, and this ratio was significantly higher in the remission group. This suggests that N-3DP alters the fatty acid composition of the cell membrane and influences clinical activity in IBD patients [41]. Although there is evidence that PUFAs can benefit IBD ex vivo and in animal models, a systematic review and meta-analyses by Turner et al. in 2011 concluded that there are insufficient data to recommend the use of omega-3 fatty acids for the maintenance of remission in CD and UC [42]. Furthermore, a systematic review in 2012 concluded that there is insufficient evidence to recommend omega-3 PUFA in IBD [43].

7. Probiotics

Probiotics have been studied extensively for inflammatory conditions, but there are few well-developed studies on probiotic use in pediatric IBD. A study by Shadnoush et al. investigated the anti-inflammatory effects of Bifidobacterium and Lactobacillus in the form of probiotic yogurt. All adult participants (210 IBD patients in remission and 95 healthy controls) were randomized to probiotic yogurt or plain yogurt. After eight weeks of oral yogurt ingestions, serum levels of IL-1β, TNF-α and CRP were significantly decreased in the probiotic yogurt group compared to their baseline values and intervention groups. The serum levels of IL-6 and IL-10 increased significantly after the intervention compared to baseline values and plain yogurt levels (all p-values < 0.05). The authors concluded that intestinal homeostasis is a balance between the pro- and anti-inflammatory responses of intestinal immunocytes and could be maintained by probiotics [44]. A small study of 21 adult UC patients by Ishikawa et al. looked at Bifidobacteria-fermented milk (BFM) for UC and concluded that supplementation with the BFM product of 100 mL per day for one year was successful in maintaining remission and had possible preventive effects on the relapse of ulcerative colitis [45]. *Lactobacillus rhamnosus* GG is a strain of *L. rhamnosus* isolated in 1983 from the intestinal tract of a healthy human which was patented by Sherwood Gorbach and Barry Goldin. A study by Zocco *et al.* investigated the efficacy of *Lactobacillus* GG in maintaining remission in 187 patients with UC. The authors compared *Lactobacillus* GG alone, *Lactobacillus* GG in combination with mesalamine and mesalamine alone. Disease activity index, endoscopic and histological scores were determined at 0, 6 and 12 months and in the case of relapse. The study showed no difference in relapse rate at 6 ($p = 0.44$) and 12 months ($p = 0.77$) among the three treatment groups. Interestingly, treatment with *Lactobacillus* GG seemed to be more effective than standard treatment with mesalazine in prolonging the relapse-free time ($p < 0.05$). *Lactobacillus* GG was found to be effective and safe for maintaining remission in patients with UC, and it may represent a good therapeutic option for preventing relapse [46].

VSL#3 is a potent probiotic composed of eight strains of lactic acid bacteria including, *S. thermophilus* MB455, *B. breve* Y8, *B. longum* Y10 (recently reclassified as *B. lactis*), *B. infantis* Y1, *L. acidophilus* MB443, *L. plantarum* MB452, *L. paracasei* MB451 and *L. bulgaricus* MB453. VSL#3 is available in a single-strength capsule containing 112.5 billion bacteria, a double strength (DS) sachet containing 900 billion bacteria and a JUNIOR packet containing 225 billion bacteria. The dosing of VSL#3 in adults with active UC is 8–16 capsules daily or 1–2 DS sachets daily. For maintenance of remission, the dose is 4–8 capsules daily or one DS sachet. For a child less than two years of age, the dose of VSL#3 for active UC is 1–3 capsules per day and for maintenance is one capsule per day. For those unable to swallow the capsule whole, the capsule may be opened and sprinkled onto a soft food or beverage. In children ages 2–5 years, for active UC, the dose of VSL#3 is 2–3 capsules or one JUNIOR packet per day, and for maintenance, it is 1–2 capsules per day. In children ages 6–11 years of age, the dose of VSL#3 in active UC is 2–4 JUNIOR packets or 4–8 capsules per day, and for maintenance, the dose is 1–2 JUNIOR packets or 2–4 capsules per day. For children ages 12–17 years, the dose of VSL#3 for active UC is 4–8 JUNIOR packets or one DS sachet per day, and for maintenance, it is 2–4 JUNIOR packets or 0.5–1 DS sachets per day. VSL#3 must be kept refrigerated to maintain its potency. VSL#3 is well tolerated. Mild abdominal bloating in the first few days of consuming VSL#3 is the most commonly reported side effect. One randomized, placebo-controlled trial in children showed the efficacy and safety of a highly concentrated mixture of VSL#3 in active UC and demonstrated its role in the maintenance of remission [47]. Similarly, a pilot study of VSL#3 in pediatric patients with mild to moderate UC showed a remission rate of 56% and a combined remission/response rate of 61% [48]. From a meta-analysis of randomized controlled trials (RCTs), administration of VSL#3 can help induce and maintain remission in UC and has been shown to maintain antibiotic-induced remission in relapsing pouchitis. The meta-analysis also concluded that other probiotics have not shown such benefit in UC nor in CD [49]. To date, the efficacy of any probiotic in the treatment of CD has not been clearly demonstrated [50,51].

8. Herbs

A number of herbs are used by IBD sufferers; however, studies of the benefits and side effects of these herbs are limited. Patients use herbs because of their perceived efficacy, safety and often low cost. Ginger (*Zingiber officinale*) is an herb that is native to Southeast Asia that has been used as a flavoring agent for more than 4,000 years. The root of the ginger plant is most useful for its anti-nausea and anti-bloating effects. Ginger can be consumed directly, as a tea or in capsule form. Caution should be taken in patients on heparin or Coumadin, as ginger may react adversely with these medications. Although ginger has not specifically been studied in pediatric IBD, children with GI symptoms, like nausea, can benefit from ginger [52]. *Boswellia serrata*, an Ayurvedic herb also known as Indian frankincense, is commonly used around the world for IBD. In adults, the *Boswellia* dosage is generally 300–400 mg three-times daily of an extract that contains 37.5% boswellic acids. In a German study of adults with IBD, 36% were taking *Boswellia serrata* extracts [53]. One study by Gupta *et al.* of 30 patients with chronic UC showed *Boswellia* to be similar to sulfasalazine in the UC remission rate. In the study, 14 of the 20 patients treated with *Boswellia* achieved remission, while four of the 10 patients treated with mesalamine achieved remission [54]. A study by Gerhardt *et al.* concluded that therapy with *Boswellia serrata* extract H15 is not inferior to mesalazine in CD [55]. The herb is well tolerated, but one study in 2011 by Holtmeier *et al.* did not find it to be superior to placebo for CD [56]. It should be noted that *Boswellia* can accelerate menstrual flow and may induce miscarriage in pregnant women. Other side effects include nausea, diarrhea and skin rashes. *Boswellia* may also decrease the anti-inflammatory effects of NSAIDs.

Oral *Aloe vera* gel is also used worldwide for IBD, because of its anti-inflammatory properties. *Aloe vera* gel comes from the inner portion of the aloe plant and is a clear, jelly-like substance. *Aloe vera* latex is yellow in color and comes from inside the outer lining of the leaf. *Aloe vera* latex is a potent laxative and should generally be avoided in UC. In active UC, oral *Aloe vera* gel taken for four weeks has been shown to produce a clinical response more often than placebo. This was studied by Langmead *et al.* in a double-blind randomized trial of 44 patients with mild to moderate active UC in which 30 patients were given 100 mL of oral *Aloe vera* gel twice daily and 14 patients were given 100 mL of placebo twice daily [57]. *Aloe vera* gel is generally well tolerated. It should be noted that oral *Aloe vera* may lower blood glucose levels, and there have been a few case reports of acute hepatitis from oral *Aloe vera* [58–59]. Although the mechanism of action of *Aloe vera* is not well understood, there are potential benefits of the herb in IBD.

Curcumin is the principal curcuminoid of the popular South Asian spice, turmeric, which is a member of the ginger family (*Zingiberaceae*). An open label pilot study in 10 adults with UC or CD documented improvement of symptoms with oral intake of 550 mg of curcumin three times a day [60]. Curcumin was shown by Hanai *et al.* to be effective for relapse prevention in adult patients with UC in a randomized, multicenter, double-blind, placebo-controlled trial [61]. A pilot pediatric study of curcumin in 11 patients showed good tolerability of the drug with only one documented side effect, gassiness, in two of the 11 patients. All participants in this pilot study received 500 mg of curcumin twice a day for three weeks, and with use of the forced-dose titration design, doses were increased up to 1 g twice a day at Week 3 for a total of three weeks and then titrated again to 2 g twice a day at Week 6 for three weeks. By using the Pediatric Crohn's Disease Activity Index (PCDAI) and Pediatric Ulcerative Colitis Activity Index (PUCAI), which are validated measures of disease activity, scores were obtained at Weeks 3, 6 and 9. Three patients saw improvement in their PCDAI/PUCAI score with the use of curcumin [62]. Curcumin is well tolerated and does not cause significant side effects. Reported side effects include stomach upset, nausea, dizziness and diarrhea. Curcumin may inhibit platelet aggregation and increase the risk of bleeding. Therefore, curcumin should be discontinued 1–2 weeks prior to any surgical procedure.

Diet with nutraceutical therapy (DNT) is a specialized therapy that is being used among IBD patients. In an uncontrolled prospective case study of six adolescent patients with CD, all six patients went into remission with discontinuation of all pharmacological drugs within two months of starting DNT. The DNT included adequate caloric and protein intake for catch-up weight gain; elimination of dairy products, certain grains and carrageenan-containing foods; nutraceuticals consisting of fish peptides, bovine colostrum, *Boswellia serrata*, curcumin and a multivitamin daily; the probiotic, *Lactobacillus* GG, twice weekly; and recombinant human GH (rhGH) daily. Three patients remained in sustained remission for four to eight years [63]. The results of this study are impressive. Further research is warranted to evaluate the efficacy of DNT among IBD patients of all ages.

Slippery elm, also known as *Ulmus fulva*, is a supplement made from the powdered bark of the slippery elm tree that is being used in IBD. Although it has not been studied in humans, an *in vitro* study by Langmead *et al.* showed that slippery elm has antioxidant effects. The study also showed that devil's claw, Mexican yam, tormentil and wei tong ning, a traditional Chinese medicine, have antioxidant properties [64]. A study in adult patients of tormentil extract (TE) showed that it can be beneficial in UC, and the herb appears to be safe in doses up to 3,000 mg per day. Interestingly, an RCT of 40 children in Russia showed that TE can shorten the duration of rotavirus diarrhea and decrease the requirement for rehydration solutions in children. Although this study was performed in children without IBD, the effects of TE may be positive on children with IBD and warrants further study. In a systematic review of 21 RCTs in 2013, for UC, *Aloe vera* gel, *Triticum aestivum* (wheat grass juice), *Andrographis paniculata* extract (HMPL-004) and topical Xilei-san were superior to placebo in inducing remission, and curcumin was superior to placebo in maintaining remission. This study also concluded that in UC, *Boswellia serrata* gum resin and *Plantago ovata* seeds were as effective as mesalamine, whereas *Oenothera biennis* (evening primrose oil) had relapse rates similar to PUFAs. The authors of the systematic review concluded that in CD, *Artemisia absinthium* (wormwood) and *Tripterygium wilfordii* were superior to placebo in inducing remission and in preventing clinical recurrence of postoperative CD, respectively [65]. Blond psyllium, glutamine and wheatgrass are other herbs used by IBD patients. Unfortunately, there is no evidence in the pediatric literature to support their use in IBD.

9. Helminthes

It is hypothesized that a lack of exposure to helminthes in the modern era of improved hygiene and healthcare has contributed to the increase of certain autoimmune conditions, like IBD. Ruyssers *et al.* noted: "Although therapy with living helminthes appears to be effective in several immunological diseases, the disadvantages of a treatment based on living parasites are explicit." [66]. An open trial in adults showed that administration of eggs from the porcine whipworm, *Trichuris suis*, to patients with CD and UC was both safe and resulted in improvement in clinical activity as measured by the Crohn's Disease Activity Index, Simple Clinical Colitis Activity Index

(SCCAI) and the Inflammatory Bowel Disease Quality of Life Index (IBDQ) [67]. To my knowledge, helminth therapy in children with IBD has not been studied.

10. Acupuncture

There is a growing body of evidence for the use of acupuncture in adults and children for a variety of diseases. In the realm of IBD, more studies are needed. One prospective, randomized, controlled clinical trial by Joos *et al.* of 29 patients with mild to moderately active UC concluded that both traditional and sham acupuncture seem to offer an added benefit in patients with active UC [68]. A second group also led by Joos *et al.* studied acupuncture in 51 patients with CD via a randomized controlled trial and showed that apart from a marked placebo effect, traditional acupuncture offers an additional therapeutic benefit in patients with mild to moderately active CD [69]. In a systematic review and meta-analysis of 43 RCTs, Ji *et al.* concluded that acupuncture and moxibustion therapy demonstrate better efficacy than oral sulfasalazine in treating IBD. However, "given the limitations of this systematic review and the included literature, definitive conclusions regarding the exact efficacy of acupuncture and moxibustion treatment for IBD cannot be drawn. Extant RCTs still cannot provide sufficient evidence and multicenter, double-blind RCTs with large sample sizes are needed to provide higher-quality evidence." [70]. Acupuncture may be beneficial for children with IBD to relieve symptoms, such as abdominal pain and nausea, but acupuncture in pediatric IBD has not been formally studied.

11. Psychological Health and Relaxation

Stress likely does not cause IBD, but stress can worsen symptoms of IBD for many patients. Using relaxation techniques, like meditation, reflexology, guided imagery and aromatherapy, may help IBD patients feel better. Pediatric patients may also find benefit from reading books and listening to music. A 2010 study examining the use of mind-body therapies in 67 adolescents reported that 62% used prayer, 40% used relaxation and 21% used imagery once/day to once/week for symptom management [71]. A Cochrane Database Review in 2012 concluded that psychological interventions, including psychotherapy, patient education and relaxation techniques, may be beneficial for adolescents with IBD, but the evidence is limited [72]. A study of 39 adults with IBD showed that those who went through a relaxation-training intervention with guided imagery showed statistically significant improvement in anxiety, mood, pain and stress compared to the control group [73]. An interesting study of female adolescents with IBD and their caregivers showed that a one-day intervention (disease-related coping skills, pain management, relaxation techniques, communication and limit setting for the parents) resulted in reduced physical symptoms and improved coping [74]. A study in the Netherlands of adolescents with IBD showed that a psychoeducational intervention can have a positive effect on coping (predictive control, $p < 0.01$), feelings of competence (global self-worth, $p < 0.05$, and physical appearance, $p < 0.01$) and health-related quality of life (body image, $p < 0.05$) [75].

Cognitive behavioral therapy has also been shown to improve global psychosocial functioning and to lessen depressive symptoms in youths with IBD [76]. A recent study by Almadani *et al.* has shown that students with IBD do not adjust to college as well as healthy students. The study used the Short Inflammatory Bowel Disease Questionnaire (SIBDQ) and showed that students with active IBD reported feeling as if they were not doing well for the amount of work they were doing, and students with ulcerative colitis reported irregular class attendance. Almadani *et al.* concluded that "Strategies to increase disease control and provide social and emotional support during college could improve adjustment to college and academic performance, and increase patients' potential." [77]. Biofeedback has been shown to improve symptoms of dyssynergic defecation, which is defined as constipation, rectal urgency/incontinence, increased stooling or rectal pain in IBD patients in remission. In a study of 30 adults with dyssynergic defecation who completed biofeedback therapy, 30% had a clinically significant improvement in quality of life as noted by the SIBDQ score and a reduction in healthcare utilization after a six-month period [78]. An interesting survey study of 27 pediatric IBD patients and one of their parents (82% mothers) has shown that parents may be good proxies for quality-of-life ratings for their children, but parents often underreport their child's health-related quality of life [79]. This suggests that parents should be encouraged to openly discuss their child's symptoms regularly. Interventions, like counseling, support groups and other available therapies, can then be initiated if needed to help a child cope with the disease.

Irritable bowel syndrome (IBS) is a disease process distinctly different from IBD. However, there may be overlap of symptoms in many patients. A study in 2002 by Simrén *et al.* investigated quality of life in IBD patients by focusing on 43 adult patients with UC and 40 with CD. All subjects had been in remission for at least one year according to laboratory parameters and clinical and endoscopical appearance. These patients completed four questionnaires evaluating GI symptoms, anxiety, depression and psychological general well-being. Thirty-three percent of UC patients and 57% of CD patients had IBS-like symptoms. The group with IBS-like symptoms (both UC and CD) had higher levels of anxiety and depression and more reduced well-being than those without. The authors concluded that "the prevalence of IBS-like symptoms in IBD patients in long-standing remission is two to three times higher than that in the normal population. Psychological factors seem to be of importance in this process. However, as a group, IBD patients in remission demonstrate psychological well-being comparable to that of the general population." [80]. There are a variety of integrative treatments available for IBS, like herbs, yoga and acupuncture, but allopathic treatment options for IBS are limited. Tricyclic antidepressants (TCAs) are commonly used to treat IBS. A study by Iskandar *et al.* of 81 IBD patients with residual gastrointestinal (GI) symptoms and 77 IBS patients showed that TCA use led to moderate improvement of residual GI symptoms in IBD patients for whom escalation of IBD therapy was not planned. UC patients demonstrated higher therapeutic success than CD patients [81]. A systematic review of 12 studies investigating antidepressants in IBD concluded that although most studies showed some benefit, there is currently insufficient data to determine the efficacy of antidepressants in IBD [82]. For practitioners, considering the overlap between IBS and IBD may help guide integrative treatment of IBD patients.

12. Clinical Hypnotherapy

According to Moser, "Gut-directed hypnotherapy (GHT) has been used successfully in functional gastrointestinal disorders. Few experimental studies and case reports have been published for IBD. GHT increases the health-related quality of life and reduces symptoms. Additionally, GHT seems to have an immune-modulating effect and is able to augment clinical remission in patients with quiescent ulcerative colitis" [83]. Well-controlled studies on clinical hypnotherapy in pediatric IBD are needed.

13. Exercise

Exercise can create a sense of well-being. However, exercise can pose challenges for patients with IBD as UC and CD often cause fatigue, abdominal pain, diarrhea and incontinence. All of these symptoms can create barriers to regular exercise. When patients are feeling well enough, they should be encouraged to engage in physical activity appropriate for age and physical fitness level. Low-impact activities, like walking, yoga and tai chi, are good options for most IBD patients. Limited evidence shows that mild to moderate exercise in adults with IBD can benefit the patient without adverse effects [84]. One study showed that lean body mass and physical activity were reduced in 39 children with IBD, whether they were in remission or in the active phase of their disease compared to 39 healthy age-matched controls [85]. As physical activity is necessary for optimal bone and muscle growth, engaging in exercise is important for pediatric IBD patients.

14. Smoking

Although it may seem simple, smoking has a complicated effect on IBD. Current smoking increases the risk of developing CD and worsens its course. On the other hand, smoking protects against UC, and in patients with UC, smoking improves its course. Smoking cessation may worsen CD, but improve UC. However, given the harmful long-term effects of smoking on the entire body, smoking cessation should be considered in all pediatric patients [86].

15. Conclusions

CAM use in IBD is prevalent and needs to be monitored and researched. As there is potential for improved quality of life and decreased need for allopathic medications with CAM, children and adolescents with IBD will continue to search for treatments that help them with their physical disease and with their ability to cope with their disease. The evidence supporting CAM in pediatrics is small, but growing. General pediatric healthcare professionals and pediatric GI specialists should respond to this trend and address CAM use in their daily practice. This initiative will result in more effective counseling for their families and more integrated care for their patients.

Acknowledgements

Thanks to the Crohn's and Colitis Foundation of America for providing support to sufferers of Crohn's disease and Ulcerative Colitis. Thanks to Mark Meyer from Baylor College of Medicine for diligently helping with this submission.

Conflicts of Interest

The author declares no conflict of interest.

References

1. Mendeloff, A.I.; Calkins, B.M. The epidemiology of idiopathic inflammatory bowel disease. In *Inflammatory Bowel Disease*; Kirsner, J.B., Shorter, R.G., Eds.; Lea & Febiger: Philadelphia, PA, USA, 1988; p. 3.
2. Van Limbergen, J.; Russell, R.K.; Drummond, H.E.; Aldhous, M.C.; Round, N.K.; Nimmo, E.R.; Smith, L.; Gillett, P.M.; McGrogan, P.; Weaver, L.T.; *et al.* Definition of phenotypic characteristics of childhood-onset inflammatory bowel disease. *Gastroenterology* **2008**, *135*, 1114–1122.
3. Vernier-Massouille, G.; Balde, M.; Salleron, J.; Turck, D.; Dupas, J.L.; Mouterde, O.; Merle, V.; Salomez, J.L.; Branche, J.; Marti, R.; *et al.* Natural history of pediatric Crohn's disease: A population-based cohort study. *Gastroenterology* **2008**, *135*, 1106–1113.
4. Roth, M.P.; Petersen, G.M.; McElree, C.; Vadheim, C.M.; Panish, J.F.; Rotter, J.I. Familial empiric risk estimates of inflammatory bowel disease in Ashkenazi Jews. *Gastroenterology* **1989**, *96*, 1016–1020.
5. Fielding, J.F. The relative risk of inflammatory bowel disease among parents and siblings of Crohn's disease patients. *J. Clin. Gastroenterol.* **1986**, *8*, 655–657.
6. Satsangi, J.; Grootscholten, C.; Holt, H.; Jewell, D.P. Clinical patterns of familial inflammatory bowel disease. *Gut* **1996**, *38*, 738–741.
7. Orholm, M.; Munkholm, P.; Langholz, E.; Nielsen, O.H.; Sørensen, T.I.; Binder, V. Familial occurrence of inflammatory bowel disease. *N. Engl. J. Med.* **1991**, *324*, 84–88.
8. Peeters, M.; Nevens, H.; Baert, F.; Hiele, M.; de Meyer, A.M.; Vlietinck, R.; Rutgeerts, P. Familial aggregation in Crohn's disease: Increased age-adjusted risk and concordance in clinical characteristics. *Gastroenterology* **1996**, *111*, 597–603.
9. Yang, H.; McElree, C.; Roth, M.P.; Shanahan, F.; Targan, S.R.; Rotter, J.I. Familial empirical risks for inflammatory bowel disease: Differences between Jews and non-Jews. *Gut* **1993**, *34*, 517–524.
10. Nunes, T.; Fiorino, G.; Danese, S.; Sans, M. Familial aggregation in inflammatory bowel disease: Is it genes or environment? *World J. Gastroenterol.* **2011**, *17*, 2715–2722.
11. Halfvarson, J.; Bodin, L.; Tysk, C.; Lindberg, E.; Järnerot, G. Inflammatory bowel disease in a Swedish twin cohort: A long-term follow-up of concordance and clinical characteristics. *Gastroenterology* **2003**, *124*, 1767–1773.

12. Thompson, N.P.; Driscoll, R.; Pounder, R.E.; Wakefield, A.J. Genetics versus environment in inflammatory bowel disease: Results of a British twin study. *BMJ* **1996**, *312*, 95–96.

13. Spehlmann, M.E.; Begun, A.Z.; Burghardt, J.; Lepage, P.; Raedler, A.; Schreiber, S. Epidemiology of inflammatory bowel disease in a German twin cohort: Results of a nationwide study. *Inflamm. Bowel Dis.* **2008**, *14*, 968–976.

14. Ananthakrishnan, A.N.; Higuchi, L.M.; Huang, E.S.; Khalili, H.; Richter, J.M.; Fuchs, C.S.; Chan, A.T. Aspirin, nonsteroidal anti-inflammatory drug use, and risk for Crohn disease and ulcerative colitis: A cohort study. *Ann. Intern. Med.* **2012**, *156*, 350–359.

15. Korelitz, B.I.; Rajapakse, R.; Schwarz, S.; Horatagis, A.P.; Gleim, G. Effects of nonsteroidal anti-inflammatory drugs on inflammatory bowel disease: A case-control study. *Am. J. Gastroenterol.* **2000**, *95*, 1949–1954.

16. Bernstein, C.N.; Singh, S.; Graff, L.A.; Walker, J.R.; Miller, N.; Cheang, M. A prospective population-based study of triggers of symptomatic flares in IBD. *Am. J. Gastroenterol.* **2010**, *105*, 1994–2002.

17. Radon, K.; Windstetter, D.; Poluda, A.L.; Mueller, B.; von Mutius, E.; Koletzko, S. Contact with farm animals in early life and juvenile inflammatory bowel disease: A case-control study. *Pediatrics* **2007**, *120*, 354–361.

18. Hlavaty, T.; Toth, J.; Koller, T.; Krajcovicova, A.; Oravcova, S.; Zelinkova, Z.; Huorka, M. Smoking, breastfeeding, physical inactivity, contact with animals, and size of the family influence the risk of inflammatory bowel disease: A Slovak case-control study. *United European Gastroenterol. J.* **2013**, *1*, 109–119.

19. Hafner, S.; Timmer, A.; Herfarth, H.; Rogler, G.; Schölmerich, J.; Schäffler, A.; Ehrenstein, B.; Jilg, W.; Ott, C.; Strauch, U.G.; *et al.* The role of domestic hygiene in inflammatory bowel diseases: Hepatitis A and worm infestations. *Eur. J. Gastroenterol. Hepatol.* **2008**, *20*, 561–566.

20. Bernstein, C.N.; Rawsthorne, P.; Cheang, M.; Blanchard, J.F. A population-based case control study of potential risk factors for IBD. *Am. J. Gastroenterol.* **2006**, *101*, 993–1002.

21. Shaw, S.Y.; Blanchard, J.F.; Bernstein, C.N. Association between the use of antibiotics in the first year of life and pediatric inflammatory bowel disease. *Am. J. Gastroenterol.* **2010**, *105*, 2687–2692.

22. Wong, A.P.; Clark, A.L.; Garnett, E.A.; Acree, M.; Cohen, S.A.; Ferry, G.D.; Heyman, M.B. Use of complementary medicine in pediatric patients with inflammatory bowel disease: Results from a multicenter survey. *J. Pediatr. Gastroenterol. Nutr.* **2009**, *48*, 55–60.

23. Day, A.S.; Whitten, K.E.; Bohane, T.D. Use of complementary and alternative medicines by children and adolescents with inflammatory bowel disease. *J. Paediatr. Child Health* **2004**, *40*, 681–684.

24. Heuschkel, R.; Afzal, N.; Wuerth, A.; Zurakowski, D.; Leichtner, A.; Kemper, K.; Tolia, V.; Bousvaros, A. Complementary medicine use in children and young adults with inflammatory bowel disease. *Am. J. Gastroenterol.* **2002**, *97*, 382–388.

25. Nousiainen, P.; Merras-Salmio, L.; Aalto, K.; Kolho, K.L. Complementary and alternative medicine use in adolescents with inflammatory bowel disease and juvenile idiopathic arthritis. *BMC Complement. Altern. Med.* **2014**, *14*, 124.

26. Koletzko, S.; Sherman, P.; Corey, M.; Griffiths, A.; Smith, C. Role of infant feeding practices in development of Crohn's disease in childhood. *BMJ* **1989**, *298*, 1617–1618.

27. Koletzko, S.; Griffiths, A.; Corey, M.; Smith, C.; Sherman, P. Infant feeding practices and ulcerative colitis in childhood. *BMJ* **1991**, *302*, 1580–1581.

28. Barclay, A.R.; Russell, R.K.; Wilson, M.L.; Gilmour, W.H.; Satsangi, J.; Wilson, D.C. Systematic review: The role of breastfeeding in the development of pediatric inflammatory bowel disease. *J. Pediatr.* **2009**, *155*, 421–426.

29. Vernia, P.; Loizos, P.; di Giuseppantonio, I.; Amore, B.; Chiappini, A.; Cannizzaro, S. Dietary calcium intake in patients with inflammatory bowel disease. *J. Crohns Colitis* **2014**, *1*, 312–317.

30. Brasil Lopes, M.; Rocha, R.; Castro Lyra, A.; Rosa Oliveira, V.; Gomes Coqueiro, F.; Silveira Almeida, N.; Santos Valois, S. Oliveira Santana GRestriction of dairy products: A reality in inflammatory bowel disease patients. *Nutr. Hosp.* **2014**, *29*, 575–581.

31. Gottschall, E. Science behind the diet. Available online: http://www.breakingtheviciouscycle.info/p/science-behind-the-diet/ (accessed on 4 August 2014).

32. Suskind, D.L.; Wahbeh, G.; Gregory, N.; Vendettuoli, H.; Christie, D. Nutritional therapy in pediatric Crohn disease: The specific carbohydrate diet. *J. Pediatr. Gastroenterol. Nutr.* **2014**, *58*, 87–91.

33. Cohen, S.A.; Gold, B.D.; Oliva, S.; Lewis, J.; Stallworth, A.; Koch, B.; Eshee, L.; Mason, D. Clinical and mucosal improvement with the specific carbohydrate diet in Pediatric Crohn's Disease: A prospective pilot study. *J. Pediatr. Gastroenterol. Nutr.* **2014**, PMID: 24897165.

34. Nahidi, L.; Day, A.S.; Lemberg, D.A.; Leach, S.T. Paediatric inflammatory bowel disease: A mechanistic approach to investigate exclusive enteral nutrition treatment. *Scientifica* **2014**, doi:10.1155/2014/423817.

35. De Bie, C.; Kindermann, A.; Escher, J. Use of exclusive enteral nutrition in paediatric Crohn's disease in The Netherlands. *J. Crohns Colitis* **2013**, *7*, 263–270.

36. Knight, C.; El-Matary, W.; Spray, C.; Sandhu, B.K. Long-term outcome of nutritional therapy in paediatric Crohn's disease. *Clin. Nutr.* **2005**, *24*, 775–779.

37. Heuschkel, R.B.; Menache, C.C.; Megerian, J.T.; Baird, A.E. Enteral nutrition and corticosteroids in the treatment of acute Crohn's disease in children. *J. Pediatr. Gastroenterol. Nutr.* **2000**, *31*, 8–15.

38. Dziechciarz, P.; Horvath, A.; Shamir, R.; Szajewska, H. Meta-analysis: Enteral nutrition in active Crohn's disease in children. *Aliment. Pharmacol. Ther.* **2007**, *26*, 795–806.

39. Sonnenberg, A. Geographic variation in the incidence of and mortality from inflammatory bowel disease. *Dis. Colon Rectum* **1986**, *29*, 854–861.

40. Socha, P.; Ryzko, J.; Koletzko, B.; Celinska-Cedro, D.; Woynarowski, M.; Czubkowski, P.; Socha, J. Essential fatty acid depletion in children with inflammatory bowel disease. *Scand. J. Gastroenterol.* **2005**, *40*, 573–577.

41. Uchiyama, K.; Nakamura, M.; Odahara, S.; Koido, S.; Katahira, K.; Shiraishi, H.; Ohkusa, T.; Fujise, K.; Tajiri, H. N-3 polyunsaturated fatty acid diet therapy for patients with inflammatory bowel disease. *Inflamm. Bowel Dis.* **2010**, *16*, 1696–1707.

42. Turner, D.; Shah, P.S.; Steinhart, A.H.; Zlotkin, S.; Griffiths, A.M. Maintenance of remission in inflammatory bowel disease using omega-3 fatty acids (fish oil): A systematic review and meta-analyses. *Inflamm. Bowel Dis.* **2011**, *17*, 336–345.

43. Cabré, E.; Mañosa, M.; Gassull, M.A. Omega-3 fatty acids and inflammatory bowel diseases—A systematic review. *Br. J. Nutr.* **2012**, *107*, S240–S252.

44. Shadnoush, M.; Shaker Hosseini, R.; Mehrabi, Y.; Delpisheh, A.; Alipoor, E.; Faghfoori, Z.; Mohammadpour, N.; Zaringhalam Moghadam, J. Probiotic yogurt affects pro- and anti-inflammatory factors in patients with inflammatory bowel disease. *Iran J. Pharm. Res.* **2013**, *12*, 929–936.

45. Ishikawa, H.; Akedo, I.; Umesaki, Y.; Tanaka, R.; Imaoka, A.; Otani, T. Randomized controlled trial of the effect of bifidobacteria-fermented milk on ulcerative colitis. *J. Am. Coll. Nutr.* **2003**, *22*, 56–63.

46. Zocco, M.A.; dal Verme, L.Z.; Cremonini, F.; Piscaglia, A.C.; Nista, E.C.; Candelli, M.; Novi, M.; Rigante, D.; Cazzato, I.A.; Ojetti, V.; *et al.* Efficacy of Lactobacillus GG in maintaining remission of ulcerative colitis. *Aliment. Pharmacol. Ther.* **2006**, *23*, 1567–1574.

47. Miele, E.; Pascarella, F.; Giannetti, E.; Quaglietta, L.; Baldassano, R.N.; Staiano, A. Effect of a probiotic preparation (VSL#3) on induction and maintenance of remission in children with ulcerative colitis. *Am. J. Gastroenterol.* **2009**, *104*, 437–443.

48. Huynh, H.Q.; deBruyn, J.; Guan, L.; Diaz, H.; Li, M.; Girgis, S.; Turner, J.; Fedorak, R.; Madsen, K. Probiotic preparation VSL#3 induces remission in children with mild to moderate acute ulcerative colitis: A pilot study. *Inflamm. Bowel Dis.* **2009**, *15*, 760–768.

49. Shen, J.; Zuo, Z.X.; Mao, A.P. Effect of probiotics on inducing remission and maintaining therapy in ulcerative colitis, Crohn's disease, and pouchitis: Meta-analysis of randomized controlled trials. *Inflamm. Bowel Dis.* **2014**, *20*, 21–35.

50. Dieleman, L.; Hoentjen, F. Probiotics have a limited role in the treatment of inflammatory bowel disease. *Ned. Tijdschr. Geneeskd.* **2012**, *156*, A5206.

51. Ruemmele, F.M.; Veres, G.; Kolho, K.L.; Griffiths, A.; Levine, A.; Escher, J.C.; Amil Dias, J.; Barabino, A.; Braegger, C.P.; Bronsky, J.; *et al.* Consensus guidelines of ECCO/ESPGHAN on the medical management of pediatric Crohn's disease. *J. Crohns Colitis* **2014**, doi:10.1016/j.crohns.2014.04.005.

52. Perez, M.E.; Youssef, N.N. Dyspepsia in childhood and adolescence: Insights and treatment considerations. *Curr. Gastroenterol. Rep.* **2007**, *9*, 447–455.

53. Joos, S.; Rosemann, T.; Szecsenyi, J.; Hahn, E.G.; Willich, S.N.; Brinkhaus, B. Use of complementary and alternative medicine in Germany—A survey of patients with inflammatory bowel disease. *BMC Complement. Altern. Med.* **2006**, *6*, 19.

54. Gupta, I.; Parihar, A.; Malhotra, P.; Singh, G.B.; Lüdtke, R.; Safayhi, H.; Ammon, H.P. Effects of Boswellia serrata gum resin in patients with ulcerative colitis. *Eur. J. Med. Res.* **1997**, *2*, 37–43.

55. Gerhardt, H.; Seifert, F.; Buvari, P.; Vogelsang, H.; Repges, R. Therapy of active Crohn disease with *Boswellia serrata* extract H 15. *Z. Gastroenterol.* **2001**, *39*, 11–17.

56. Holtmeier, W.; Zeuzem, S.; Preiss, J.; Kruis, W.; Böhm, S.; Maaser, C.; Raedler, A.; Schmidt, C.; Schnitker, J.; Schwarz, J.; *et al.* Randomized, placebo-controlled, double-blind trial of *Boswellia serrata* in maintaining remission of Crohn's disease: Good safety profile but lack of efficacy. *Inflamm. Bowel Dis.* **2011**, *17*, 573–582.

57. Langmead, L.; Feakins, R.M.; Goldthorpe, S.; Holt, H.; Tsironi, E.; de Silva, A.; Jewell, D.P.; Rampton, D.S. Randomized, double-blind, placebo-controlled trial of oral *aloe vera* gel for active ulcerative colitis. *Aliment. Pharmacol. Ther.* **2004**, *19*, 739–747.

58. Choudhary, M.; Kochhar, A.; Sangha, J. Hypoglycemic and hypolipidemic effect of *Aloe vera* L. in non-insulin dependent diabetics. *J. Food Sci. Technol.* **2014**, *51*, 90–96.

59. Yang, H.N.; Kim, D.J.; Kim, Y.M.; Kim, B.H.; Sohn, K.M.; Choi, M.J.; Choi, Y.H. *Aloe*-induced toxic hepatitis. *J. Korean Med. Sci.* **2010**, *25*, 492–495.

60. Holt, P.R.; Katz, S.; Kirshoff, R. Curcumin therapy in inflammatory bowel disease: A pilot study. *Dig. Dis. Sci.* **2005**, *50*, 2191–2193.

61. Hanai, H.; Iida, T.; Takeuchi, K.; Watanabe, F.; Maruyama, Y.; Andoh, A.; Tsujikawa, T.; Fujiyama, Y.; Mitsuyama, K.; Sata, M.; *et al.* Curcumin maintenance therapy for ulcerative colitis: Randomized, multicenter, double-blind, placebo-controlled trial. *Clin. Gastroenterol. Hepatol.* **2006**, *4*, 1502–1506.

62. Suskind, D.L.; Wahbeh, G.; Burpee, T.; Cohen, M.; Christie, D.; Weber, W. Tolerability of curcumin in pediatric inflammatory bowel disease: A forced-dose titration study. *J. Pediatr. Gastroenterol. Nutr.* **2013**, *56*, 277–279.

63. Slonim, A.E.; Grovit, M.; Bulone, L. Effect of exclusion diet with nutraceutical therapy in juvenile Crohn's disease. *J. Am. Coll. Nutr.* **2009**, *28*, 277–285.

64. Langmead, L.; Dawson, C.; Hawkins, C.; Banna, N.; Loo, S.; Rampton, D.S. Antioxidant effects of herbal therapies used by patients with inflammatory bowel disease: An *in vitro* study. *Aliment. Pharmacol. Ther.* **2002**, *16*, 197–205.

65. Ng, S.C.; Lam, Y.T.; Tsoi, K.K.; Chan, F.K.; Sung, J.J.; Wu, J.C. Systematic review: The efficacy of herbal therapy in inflammatory bowel disease. *Aliment. Pharmacol. Ther.* **2013**, *38*, 854–863.

66. Ruyssers, N.E.; de Winter, B.Y.; de Man, J.G.; Loukas, A.; Herman, A.G.; Pelckmans, P.A.; Moreels, T.G. Worms and the treatment of inflammatory bowel disease: Are molecules the answer? *Clin. Dev. Immunol.* **2008**, doi:10.1155/2008/567314.

67. Summers, R.W.; Elliott, D.E.; Qadir, K.; Urban, J.F., Jr.; Thompson, R.; Weinstock, J.V. Trichuris suis seems to be safe and possibly effective in the treatment of inflammatory bowel disease. *Am. J. Gastroenterol.* **2003**, *98*, 2034–2041.

68. Joos, S.; Wildau, N.; Kohnen, R.; Szecsenyi, J.; Schuppan, D.; Willich, S.N.; Hahn, E.G.; Brinkhaus, B. Acupuncture and moxibustion in the treatment of ulcerative colitis: A randomized controlled study. *Scand. J. Gastroenterol.* **2006**, *41*, 1056–1063.

69. Joos, S.; Brinkhaus, B.; Maluche, C.; Maupai, N.; Kohnen, R.; Kraehmer, N.; Hahn, E.G.; Schuppan, D. Acupuncture and moxibustion in the treatment of active Crohn's disease: A randomized controlled study. *Digestion* **2004**, *69*, 131–139.
70. Ji, J.; Lu, Y.; Liu, H.; Feng, H.; Zhang, F.; Wu, L.; Cui, Y.; Wu, H. Acupuncture and moxibustion for inflammatory bowel diseases: A systematic review and meta-analysis of randomized controlled trials. *Evid. Based Complement. Alternat. Med.* **2013**, *2013*, 158352.
71. Cotton, S.; Humenay Roberts, Y.; Tsevat, J.; Britto, M.T.; Succop, P.; McGrady, M.E.; Yi, M.S. Mind-body complementary alternative medicine use and quality of life in adolescents with inflammatory bowel disease. *Inflamm. Bowel Dis.* **2010**, *16*, 501–506.
72. Timmer, A.; Preiss, J.C.; Motschall, E.; Rücker, G.; Jantschek, G.; Moser, G. Psychological interventions for treatment of inflammatory bowel disease. *Cochrane Database Syst. Rev.* **2011**, doi:10.1002/14651858.CD006913.pub2.
73. Mizrahi, M.C.; Reicher-Atir, R.; Levy, S.; Haramati, S.; Wengrower, D.; Israeli, E.; Goldin, E. Effects of guided imagery with relaxation training on anxiety and quality of life among patients with inflammatory bowel disease. *Psychol. Health* **2012**, *27*, 1463–1479.
74. McCormick, M.; Reed-Knight, B.; Lewis, J.D.; Gold, B.D.; Blount, R.L. Coping skills for reducing pain and somatic symptoms in adolescents with IBD. *Inflamm. Bowel Dis.* **2010**, *16*, 2148–2157.
75. Grootenhuis, M.A.; Maurice-Stam, H.; Derkx, B.H.; Last, B.F. Evaluation of a psychoeducational intervention for adolescents with inflammatory bowel disease. *Eur. J. Gastroenterol. Hepatol.* **2009**, *21*, 430–435.
76. Thompson, R.D.; Craig, A.; Crawford, E.A.; Fairclough, D.; Gonzalez-Heydrich, J.; Bousvaros, A.; Noll, R.B.; DeMaso, D.R.; Szigethy, E. Longitudinal results of cognitive behavioral treatment for youths with inflammatory bowel disease and depressive symptoms. *J. Clin. Psychol. Med. Settings* **2012**, *19*, 329–337.
77. Almadani, S.B.; Adler, J.; Browning, J.; Green, E.H.; Helvie, K.; Rizk, R.S. Zimmermann EM effects of inflammatory bowel disease on students' adjustment to college. *Clin. Gastroenterol. Hepatol.* **2014**, doi:10.1016/j.cgh.2014.03.032.
78. Jowett, S.L.; Seal, C.J.; Barton, J.R.; Welfare, M.R. The short inflammatory bowel disease questionnaire is reliable and responsive to clinically important change in ulcerative colitis. *Am. J. Gastroenterol.* **2001**, *96*, 2921–2928.
79. Gallo, J.; Grant, A.; Otley, A.R.; Orsi, M.; MacIntyre, B.; Gauvry, S.; Lifschitz, C. Do parents and children agree? Quality-of-life assessment of children with inflammatory bowel disease and their parents. *J. Pediatr. Gastroenterol. Nutr.* **2014**, *58*, 481–485.
80. Simrén, M.; Axelsson, J.; Gillberg, R.; Abrahamsson, H.; Svedlund, J.; Björnsson, E.S. Quality of life in inflammatory bowel disease in remission: The impact of IBS-like symptoms and associated psychological factors. *Am. J. Gastroenterol.* **2002**, *97*, 389–396.
81. Iskandar, H.N.; Cassell, B.; Kanuri, N.; Gyawali, C.P.; Gutierrez, A.; Dassopoulos, T.; Ciorba, M.A.; Sayuk, G.S. Tricyclic antidepressants for management of residual symptoms in inflammatory bowel disease. *J. Clin. Gastroenterol.* **2014**, *48*, 423–429.

82. Mikocka-Walus, A.A.; Turnbull, D.A.; Moulding, N.T.; Wilson, I.G.; Andrews, J.M.; Holtmann, G.J. Antidepressants and inflammatory bowel disease: A systematic review. *Clin. Pract. Epidemiol. Ment. Health* **2006**, *2*, 1–9.

83. Moser, G. The role of hypnotherapy for the treatment of inflammatory bowel diseases. *Expert Rev. Gastroenterol. Hepatol.* **2014**, *8*, 601–606.

84. Nathan, I.; Norton, C.; Czuber-Dochan, W.; Forbes, A. Exercise in individuals with inflammatory bowel disease. *Gastroenterol. Nurs.* **2013**, *36*, 437–442.

85. Werkstetter, K.J.; Ullrich, J.; Schatz, S.B.; Prell, C.; Koletzko, B.; Koletzko, S. Lean body mass, physical activity and quality of life in paediatric patients with inflammatory bowel disease and in healthy controls. *J. Crohns Colitis* **2012**, *6*, 665–673.

86. Cosnes, J. Smoking, physical activity, nutrition and lifestyle: Environmental factors and their impact on IBD. *Dig. Dis.* **2010**, *28*, 411–417.

Acupuncture for Pediatric Pain

Brenda Golianu, Ann Ming Yeh and Meredith Brooks

Abstract: Chronic pain is a growing problem in children, with prevalence as high as 30.8%. Acupuncture has been found to be useful in many chronic pain conditions, and may be of clinical value in a multidisciplinary treatment program. The basic principles of acupuncture are reviewed, as well as studies exploring basic mechanisms of acupuncture and clinical efficacy. Conditions commonly treated in the pediatric pain clinic, including headache, abdominal pain, fibromyalgia, juvenile arthritis, complex regional pain syndrome, cancer pain, as well as perioperative pain studies are reviewed and discussed. Areas in need of further research are identified, and procedural aspects of acupuncture practice and safety studies are reviewed. Acupuncture can be an effective adjuvant in the care of pediatric patients with painful conditions, both in a chronic and an acute setting. Further studies, including randomized controlled trials, as well as trials of comparative effectiveness are needed.

Reprinted from *Children*. Cite as: Ruckenstein, M. Acupuncture for Pediatric Pain. *Children* **2014**, *1*, 134-148.

1. Introduction

Chronic pain is a growing problem in children with prevalence as high as 30.8% in some epidemiological studies [1]. The predominant types of pain include headache (60.8%), abdominal pain (43.3%), limb (33.6%), and back (30.2%), and pain symptoms have been found to be associated with many lifestyle restrictions including sleep problems, inability to pursue hobbies, school absences, and inability to meet with friends. Pediatric pain clinics offer many integrative and complementary services including biofeedback (33%), acupuncture (24%), massage (20%), gratitude journals (16%), yoga and tai chi (8%) [2]. In other studies of pediatric headache conducted in Italy and Germany, Complementary Alternative Medicine (CAM) therapies were utilized by 76% and 75.7% of patients respectively [3,4]. Thus, a thorough understanding of the basis and efficacy of these therapies is warranted to help our patients better navigate the extensive selection of therapies, as well as integrate them with conventional medical treatment strategies.

2. Physiology of Chronic Pain

The physiology of chronic pain has evolved from a direct stimulus response model to one of an integrated complex neural network response. Following tissue injury, there is an immediate release of local inflammatory mediators, including prostaglandins, histamine, bradykinin and other factors, which lead to a localized tissue response, consisting of localized swelling, pain, and edema. Furthermore, they sensitize the primary neurons such that a subsequent stimulus is perceived as even more painful. The development of chronic pain involves long term potentiation of peripheral nerves, molecular changes in the spinal cord and central nervous system, [5] as well as alteration in how various areas of the mid brain and limbic system, including structures such as insula, prefrontal cortex, anterior cingulate, thalamus, often termed the "pain matrix", connect to one another. These changes can be observed using functional MRI studies. Improvement in pain is often correlated with the return of normalized connectivity in these areas [6,7].

3. Acupuncture: Introduction, Mechanisms of Action, and Clinical Research

3.1. Introduction

Acupuncture has been practiced in China for at least 3000 years. The basic principles of acupuncture revolve around the concept of "Qi", or energy of the body. When this energy is not flowing correctly, it is believed to lead to illness and disease. In the traditional setting acupuncture is frequently utilized as a preventative therapy or an intervention early in the course of illness.

In the pediatric population, standard medical therapies for chronic pain conditions often carry a significant side effect profile. Side effects of frequently used pharmacological agents for chronic pain include sedation, dizziness, tolerance, nausea, constipation, as well as depression and suicidal ideation. As a result, many parents and children are especially interested in trying acupuncture and other CAM therapies due to their relatively low risk profile.

3.2. Acupuncture Mechanisms of Action

A challenging area of research has involved understanding the mechanisms of acupuncture action and how it relates to pain. Although much research has been performed in the last several decades and many basic scientific studies have outlined various physiologic pathways which are activated by acupuncture, a complete synthesis of the mechanism of action of acupuncture is still elusive [8]. Many areas of active research can be identified, and within each hundreds of studies are found, however we will mention three theories that are particularly noteworthy regarding the mechanisms of action of acupuncture: molecular mechanisms, physiologic changes found at acupuncture point locations, and central nervous system changes in brain connectivity. Principal among the molecular studies is the work of JS Han and colleagues, who over several decades explored how acupuncture stimulated the release of endogenous endorphins [9]. One of their most significant findings is that low frequency (2–10 Hz) electrical stimulation of acupuncture points leads to increased endorphin release, while high frequency stimulation (100 Hz) leads to increased dynorphin release. Other studies describe the local changes found at acupuncture points, including connective tissue changes, and changes in electrical resistance at acupoints. For example, Langevin identified changes in connective tissue that occur with the physical act of needle placement [10], while Anh *et al.* explored the changes in skin resistance at distal acupuncture points and found that changes in these responses correlated with clinical response in adolescent girls with pelvic pain [11].

A number of fMRI studies have shown changes in brain blood flow following acupuncture treatment, and normalization of activity in areas of the limbic system, as well as areas of the "pain matrix" [12–14]. An excellent review of acupuncture basic mechanisms was performed by Wang *et al.* [15].

3.3. Challenges in Acupuncture Clinical Research

In 1997, the NIH conducted a Consensus meeting, where it was determined that sufficient evidence was present to conclude that acupuncture is effective for a number of conditions including nausea and vomiting related to chemotherapy, adult postoperative pain and postoperative dental pain. Additional promising indications included tennis elbow, dysmenorrhea, stroke rehabilitation, and the treatment of addiction [16]. Since that time many additional studies have supported the use of acupuncture in a number of types of painful conditions [17,18].

Some studies, such as the back pain trial in Germany, showed an improvement in both the active and the sham acupuncture arms as compared to standard care, suggesting that some of the acupuncture effect may not depend on the specificity of the points utilized [19]. There is significant controversy in the acupuncture literature about how this matter should be interpreted, as the sham controls in many studies have shown clinical efficacy. One explanation is that since we do not know the exact mechanisms of pain relief of acupuncture, the sham controls, which involve active needle placement in alternate locations, are themselves having a therapeutic benefit. Secondly, the active acupuncture treatment that is performed as part of an RCT may have limitations, as it does not allow individualization of treatment, a necessary ingredient of acupuncture therapy. Thus the finding in many studies that active acupuncture and sham acupuncture appear to both be efficacious remains an interpretive challenge in current acupuncture research, and until this phenomenon is better understood and an appropriate, therapeutically inactive but believable sham treatment can be designed, there has been a call for different types of studies, such as comparative effectiveness trials, which compare the acupuncture therapy against standard therapies, to continue to inform clinical practice [20]. MacPherson *et al.*, in a meta-analysis of published studies, determined that positive trials were associated with more needles and more frequent treatments, suggesting that dosing of acupuncture may also be important [21].

4. Pediatric Pain

Acupuncture can be a useful adjuvant in the care of pediatric patients with painful conditions, both in the chronic and acute setting. In a study on the feasibility of acupuncture/hypnosis intervention, 33 children were offered acupuncture together with a hypnosis session while needles were in place. Treatments were highly acceptable (only 2 patients refused). Both parents and children reported decrease in pain (4.38 ($p < 0.0001$)), and improvement in function (2.62 ($p = 0.014$)) [22]. Lin *et al.* investigated the efficacy of acupuncture for children and adolescents with chronic pain. Fifty-three patients between 2 and 18 years of age, with a variety of painful conditions underwent pain assessment before and after acupuncture treatment. The average duration of pain improvement was 3 days, suggesting that continued acupuncture was needed for longer term improvement [23].

Conditions commonly treated in pediatric pain, including headache, abdominal pain, fibromyalgia, juvenile arthritis, complex regional pain syndrome, cancer pain, as well as perioperative pain studies will be discussed. Due to the paucity of acupuncture research in the pediatric literature, adult studies will also be reviewed in each section, as they often serve as the clinical basis for the development of treatment regimens. Lastly, areas in need of further research of acupuncture in children will be identified.

4.1. Procedure Consent, Acceptance and Safety of Acupuncture

4.1.1. The Procedure of Acupuncture

Informed consent is obtained from the parents prior to initiation of acupuncture treatment. The type of acupuncture is explained to both the parent and child, along with possible complications, which may include bleeding, infection, or increased pain. More serious complications have occurred (see below) and may be related to needling technique or patient condition. A refusal of the parent or child to receive acupuncture should be a contraindication. Pediatric patients often require more gentle introduction to the needling process, to allow them to grow more accustomed to the idea, trust the practitioner, and observe for themselves that the needles usually do not cause excessive discomfort. Lin *et al.* showed that while 53% of children were initially apprehensive of acupuncture needles, following their first needle 64% felt it did not hurt, and furthermore would recommend it to someone else.. Acupuncture treatment will usually consist of a series of treatments, usually 6–10, to determine if acupuncture intervention is helpful for the patient's condition. In a study by Kemper of adolescents receiving acupuncture for their pain, 67% reported the therapy as pleasant, and 70% reported that it had helped their pain [24]. Children were moderately receptive to acupuncture therapy for their chronic pain symptoms [25]. Parental experience with acupuncture, regardless of its perceived efficacy, appears to play in a role in parents' consideration of acupuncture for their child [26]. Parental stress was found to decrease along with child discomfort following acupuncture therapy for the child [27].

4.1.2. Acupuncture Safety

In an excellent review of the safety of acupuncture in the pediatric population, Adams *et al.* screened a total of 9537 references, and identified 37 studies in the international literature that satisfied criteria for inclusion. Described complications included infection, and 1 case each of cardiac rupture, pneumothorax, and other effects, likely related to direct needle organ penetration. Additional mild adverse effects included pain, bruising, and worsening of symptoms. The study concluded that acupuncture is safe when performed by appropriately trained practitioners [28]. Yates *et al.* showed that non-invasive electrical stimulation at acupuncture points during a routine heel stick was well tolerated in healthy neonates [29].

4.1.3. Headache

In the adult literature, several studies examine acupuncture as a prophylactic treatment. Allais *et al.* performed a randomized trial of 160 women migraine sufferers who received weekly acupuncture for 2 months, followed by monthly acupuncture for an additional 4 months. Decreased headache severity, as well as decreased medication usage, was statistically significant at all time points analyzed [30]. Diener *et al.* performed a large multicentre randomized study of 443 patients randomized into three groups—verum acupuncture, sham acupuncture (termed New Western acupuncture by the researchers), and standard medical care. Following 10 weekly acupuncture treatments, headache frequency and severity was measured at 26 weeks after baseline. Although the results were statistically significant, the effect size may have been diminished by the long time lapse between last acupuncture treatment and pain assessment [31]. In another study of migraine sufferers, the study intervention was delivered in a standard clinical format, without randomization. Study results showed that acupuncture had a measurable clinical effect, which was greater than that seen in a randomized format [32]. Finally two large Cochrane Collaboration Reviews concluded that although it appeared that specific point selection was not as important as had previously thought, acupuncture should be considered as a treatment option for patients needing prophylactic treatment for migraine or tension headaches [33,34].

In the pediatric population, a randomized trial of 22 children with migraine showed in the true acupuncture group the migraine frequency decreased from 9.3 ($\pm$1.6) to 1.4 ($\pm$0.6), and intensity decreased from 8.7 ($\pm$0.4) to 7.8 ($\pm$0.6) following 10 weekly sessions [35]. Gottschling *et al.* used a non-invasive technique, laser acupuncture, in a randomized trial of 43 children with either migraine or tension type headache. The mean number of headaches per month decreased by 6.4 days in the treatment group, and by 1.0 day in the placebo group ($p < 0.001$). Secondary outcomes of headache severity were likewise decreased, and were statistically significant at all time points [36]. Further studies are needed exploring the use of acupuncture as a prophylactic agent in the pediatric population, as well as studies which combine the use of a low dose prophylactic medication together with acupuncture.

4.1.4. Abdominal Pain

Abdominal pain can be due to a multitude of diagnoses, and a full review of these is beyond the scope of this work. We will first review the available adult literature on the use of acupuncture in the management of pain related to irritable bowel syndrome (IBS), a functional disorder characterized by chronic or recurrent abdominal pain or discomfort which is associated with disturbed bowel function, and feelings of abdominal distention and bloating [37]. Chao *et al.* performed a meta-analysis of 6 randomized placebo controlled studies [38]. Although five of the studies did not show statistically significant improvement, the one positive study in the group was a relatively large study [39], and thus the overall meta-analysis provided support for the use of acupuncture. A Cochrane review of acupuncture for IBS showed no benefit from acupuncture as compared to credible sham controlled therapies, however a comparative effectiveness trial of acupuncture compared to two antispasmodics (pinaverium bromide and trimebutin maleate) showed acupuncture as more effective than these standard therapies for IBS [40]. In a pediatric trial on children with intermittent abdominal pain that compared hand acupuncture to no treatment, hand acupuncture was shown to be effective [41]. As the trial was not blinded, however, the results are difficult to interpret. Further studies are needed to delineate whether there is clinical benefit of acupuncture in this condition, the necessary dose or frequency and duration of acupuncture treatment required, as well as possible mechanisms of action.

4.1.5. Pediatric Fibromyalgia

Pediatric fibromyalgia is a poorly understood condition that affects 1%–6% of populations studied, and includes symptoms of general fatigue, disordered sleep, severe myofascial pain, and abdominal dysregulation [42]. The mechanisms of fibromyalgia pain are not fully understood, but may include genetic, anatomic, metabolic and psychosocial factors [43]. Acupuncture was found to change cortical responses to painful stimuli in fibromyalgia patients, suggesting a complex inhibitory modulation may be active in the central nervous system in fibromyalgia patients [44].

In the adult population, acupuncture studies have demonstrated that acupuncture may be a significant adjunct in the care of fibromyalgia patients, and is superior to standard care alone [45]. It is noted however that sham acupuncture likewise appeared more effective than standard care, making it difficult to determine the specificity of the acupuncture needle placement in this study. Although acupuncture is routinely offered and utilized as a CAM therapy in pediatric pain clinics by patients with fibromyalgia, to date there have been no randomized controlled studies in the pediatric population [46]. Future acupuncture research in children with fibromyalgia should examine its benefits, comparative effectiveness, mechanism of action and necessary dose.

4.1.6. Acupuncture for Juvenile Arthritis

Children with juvenile idiopathic arthritis (JIA) and other rheumatological conditions utilize CAM therapies regularly, with frequencies between 34% and 92% [47]. Factors associated with CAM use include longer disease duration, presence of more than one illness, previous CAM use by parents themselves, and parents' perception that medications are not helping [48,49]. In adults, Berman *et al.*, in a landmark randomized controlled study of osteoarthritis, found that the true acupuncture group experienced a greater improvement in WOMAC function at 8 weeks than the sham acupuncture group [50]; however, a subsequent meta-analysis of nine studies showed short-term benefits compared to sham, and clinically relevant benefits relative to wait-list control [51]. Zanette *et al.* studied 40 adults on a stable medication regimen with uncontrolled rheumatoid arthritis in a randomized controlled study. There was significant improvement in patient and physician global assessment and in physician assessment of disease activity in the acupuncture group, however the primary outcome of 20% improvement in ACR criteria was not statistically significant [52]. There are no studies in the literature evaluating the effect of acupuncture on juvenile arthritis. Studies are needed to explore the efficacy of acupuncture in pediatric rheumatological conditions.

4.1.7. Pelvic Pain

Acupuncture has been shown to be effective in pain related to dysmenorrhea in multiple adult randomized clinical trials. Kiran *et al.* showed that acupuncture was as effective as NSAIDS in a small, randomized trial [53]. A Cochrane review concluded that acupuncture may be effective for dymenorrhea, however more studies were needed [54]. A study of acupressure in adolescents with dysmenorrhea showed a decrease in pain in the experimental group that was statistically significant ($p < 0.002$) compared to the sham acupressure group [55]. Sham acupressure also had some effect of improved analgesia, however, thus a third control of standard care or other relatively inert control would have been beneficial and may have shown an even greater clinical significance. In a small randomized sham controlled pediatric study on pelvic pain due to endometriosis, Wayne *et al.* showed that participants experienced a 4.8 (SD 2.4) point reduction on a 11 point scale after 4 weeks, which differed significantly from the control group who experienced an average reduction of 1.4 (SD2.1) (p = 0.004). Reduction in pain persisted 6 months after intervention; however, after 4 weeks the differences were not clinically significant, suggesting continued acupuncture may be needed for a more prolonged therapeutic effect [56]. Further research is needed in pediatric patients with pelvic pain focusing on comparative effectiveness with standard treatments, dose efficacy and mechanism of action.

4.1.8. Complex Regional Pain Syndrome

Little information exists regarding the treatment of Complex Regional Pain Syndrome (CRPS) with acupuncture. Several case reports in adult military personnel showed benefits in shoulder and hand CRPS following scalp acupuncture [57]. An adult case study involving laser acupuncture and small subcutaneous needles also proved to be effective [58]. In children, one case study describes the use of electrical stimulation at acupuncture points, while another describes the use of acupuncture in three pediatric patients leading to clinical improvement [59,60]. Further studies in children with complex regional pain syndrome, including scalp acupuncture, electrical stimulation and other specific protocols are needed to delineate whether there is measurable and reproducible benefit.

4.1.9. Acupuncture for Cancer Pain

The management of cancer pain presents a complex challenge for the oncologist and the pain practitioner. Pain may be due to acute tissue invasion, inflammation, bone pain, neuropathic pain, or a combination of causes [61]. In addition, cancer patients suffer from other chemotherapeutic side effects including nausea and vomiting. CAM therapies are frequently utilized by this population. A prevalence study of CAM use in children and adolescents with cancer in Germany found that 29% of children and 36% of adolescents used CAM therapies. Reasons for using CAM included strengthening the immune system, reduction of therapy-related side effects, and desire to increase healing chances [62]. Acupuncture was used by 12% of children and 17% of adolescents. In a randomized trial of acupuncture to alleviate chemotherapy related nausea and vomiting due to highly emetogenic chemotherapy, the need for rescue anti-emetics was significantly lower in the acupuncture group than in the control group (p < 0.001) [63]. Episodes of vomiting were likewise lower in the treatment group (p = 0.01). Acupuncture was found to be safe in patients with thrombocytopenia due to chemotherapy [64].

4.1.10. Acupuncture for Acute Pain

Two studies have explored the use of acupuncture in the treatment of acute post-operative pain in pediatric patients. Wu *et al.* reported a case series of 20 pediatric patients, aged 7 months to 18 years, who had undergone various surgeries [65]. Acupuncture was performed in the post-operative period. Pain scores declined immediately following acupuncture, as well as at 24 hours after acupuncture was performed. The acupuncture was well tolerated, and 85% of parents reported they would pay for acupuncture "out of pocket" if not covered by insurance. This study was not controlled, however.

Lin *et al.* performed a randomized trial examining pain and delirium in pediatric patients following tympanostomy surgery [66]. Sixty children were randomized to acupuncture or sham acupuncture following induction of anesthesia. Statistical differences in pain scores were observed in post anesthesia care unit at each five minute time point. Median pain scores were between 2 and 4 points lower than the sham acupuncture group. Postoperative agitation was also decreased, and showed statistical significance at all time points. Additional studies are needed to explore the magnitude of the clinical effect of various acupuncture treatments, duration of action, as well as post-operative opioid use and surgical recovery time.

4.1.11. Acupuncture for Delirium, Agitation, Withdrawal and Emotional Conditions

Several studies exist on the use of acupuncture on post-traumatic stress disorder. Hollifield *et al.* found that acupuncture was as effective as cognitive behavioral therapy, and Zhang *et al.* found that acupoint stimulation together with cognitive behavioral therapy was more effective than cognitive behavioral therapy alone [67,68]. To date, no studies have been identified examining the efficacy of acupuncture in children with post traumatic stress disorder. Several studies specifically address the effect of acupuncture interventions on withdrawal and agitation in children. Wang *et al.* found that acupressure reduced anxiety in children undergoing anesthesia [69]. Kundu *et al.* performed a retrospective review of pediatric patients who had postoperative agitation on a previous anesthetic, and received acupuncture with a subsequent anesthetic [70]. 10 patients (83%) did not exhibit symptoms of agitation, while 2 (17%) exhibited milder symptoms but were able to communicate their distress. In a study of neonates with Neonatal Abstinence Syndrome (NAS), the addition of auricular acupressure beads did not result in a different clinical course, though there was a suggestive trend toward less pharmacological support in the acupressure group [71].

4.1.12. Non-Invasive Transcutaneous Electrical Acupoint Stimulation (TEAS)

As some pediatric patients, as well as some adults, may have a fear of needles, the use of transcutaneous electric acupoint stimulation (TEAS) may provide an alternative to conventional acupuncture treatments. The effectiveness of TENS may be mediated by alpha 2A adrenergic receptors [72]. A number of studies suggest that such stimulation may be clinically effective. Wang *et al.* showed that TEAS reduced intraoperative remifentanil consumption and alleviated post-operative side effects following sinusotomy [73]. TEAS was also applied by Kabalak for the management of postoperative vomiting following tonsillectomy in children in a randomized study [74]. In another randomized double blinded perioperative study, TEAS was applied at the start of surgery in patients undergoing pediatric cardiac surgery [75]. Duration of ventilation, and length of stay in ICU were significantly lower in the active treatment group. In addition, cardiac troponin, a measure of damaged cardiac tissue, was significantly lower in the active treatment group. As TEAS is a non-invasive technique, it has significant promise as a potential treatment in children.

4.1.13. Non-Invasive Laser Acupuncture

Laser acupuncture may also be utilized in the clinic for management of pain and discomfort in the pediatric patient. In addition to the headache study as mentioned above by Gottschling *et al.*, others have demonstrated clinical utility. Ferreira *et al.* described a case report of improved trismus as a sequelae of medulobastoma in a child [76]. Other non-invasive therapies offered in pediatric pain clinics include moxibustion, cupping and acupressure magnets [77].

4.2. Cost-Effectiveness of Acupuncture Therapy

This is a relatively new area of research, however, an National Health Service (NHS) analysis of low back pain studied in 239 patients, with 159 randomized to acupuncture and 80 to usual care, found that the addition of acupuncture to standard care led to improved pain both immediately after the treatments as well as at 24 months. Though the cost of delivering acupuncture in addition to standard care was an increase of expenditure, this cost was more than balanced by a reduction in lost days of work, and decreased medical spending in other areas including hospitalization, general practitioner or other outpatient visits. This suggests an overall societal benefit to supporting the provision of acupuncture services [77]. Further research is needed examining the cost-effectiveness of acupuncture in children in relation to lost parental work days, cost of medications, and other therapeutic interventions.

5. Conclusions

Acupuncture techniques, both invasive and noninvasive, can be an important adjuvant in the care of the pediatric patient with chronic pain. Acupuncture should be performed by a trained professional, and should be incorporated in a multidisciplinary program of treatment, after appropriate workup has been performed. The evidence suggests that it is a safe and cost-effective treatment modality for pediatric pain. Further research is needed regarding the specific and non-specific effects of acupuncture, as well as mechanisms of action, dosing and frequency related to various painful conditions in pediatric patients.

Acknowledgments

The authors wish to thank their respective Departments for continued support and encouragement in the investigation of the efficacy and mechanisms of action of acupuncture therapy.

Author Contributions

Brenda Golianu contributed to the writing and editing of the manuscript. Ann Ming Yeh contributed to the writing and editing of the manuscript. Meredith Brooks contributed to the writing and editing of the manuscript.

Conflicts of Interest

The authors declare no conflict of interest.

References

1. Roth-Isigkeit, A.; Thyen, U.; Stoven, H.; Schwarzenberger, J.; Schmucker, P. Pain among children and adolescents: Restrictions in daily living and triggering factors. *Pediatrics* **2005**, *2*, e152–e162.
2. Young, L.; Kemper, K.J. Integrative care for pediatric patients with pain. *J. Altern. Complement. Med.* **2013**, *19*, 627–632.
3. Dallara Libera, D.; Colombo, B.; Pavan, G.; Comi, G. Complementary and alternative medicine (CAM) use in an Italian cohort of pediatric headache patients: The tip of the iceberg. *Neurol. Sci.* **2014**, *35*, 145–148.
4. Schetzek, S.; Heinen, F.; Kruse, S.; Borggraefe, I.; Bonfert, M.; Gaul, C.; Gottschling, S.; Ebinger, F. Headache in children: Update on complementary treatments. *Neuropediatrics* **2013**, *44*, 25–33.
5. Basbaum, A.I.; Bautista, D.M.; Scherrer, G.; Julius, D. Cellular and molecular mechanisms of pain. *Cell* **2009**, *139*, 267–284.
6. Woolf, C.J. Pain: Metabolites, mambas and mutations. *Lancet Neurol.* **2013**, *12*, 18–19.
7. Baliki, M.N.; Petre, B.; Torbey, S.; Herrmann, K.M.; Huang, L.; Schnitzer, T.J.; Fields, H.L.; Apkarian, A.V. Corticostriatal functional connectivity predicts transition to chronic back pain. *Nat. Neurosci.* **2012**, *15*, 1117–1119.
8. Napadow, V.; Anh, A.; Longhurst, J.; Lao, L.; Stener-Victorin, E.; Harris, R.; Langevin, H.M. The status and future of acupuncture mechanism research. *J. Altern. Complement. Med.* **2008**, *14*, 861–869.
9. Han, J.S. Acupuncture: Neuropeptide release produced by electrical stimulation of different frequencies. *Trends Neurosci.* **2003**, *26*, 17–22.
10. Langevin, H.M.; Bouffard, N.A.; Churchill, D.L.; Badger, G.J. Connective tissue fibroblast response to acupuncture: Dose-dependent effect of bidirectional needle rotation. *J. Altern. Complement. Med.* **2007**, *13*, 355–360.
11. Ahn, A.C.; Schnyer, R.; Conboy, L.; Laufer, M.R.; Wayne, P.M. Electrodermal measures of jing-well points and their clinical relevance in endometriosis-related chronic pelvic pain. *J. Altern. Complement. Med.* **2009**, *15*, 1293–1305.
12. Hui, K.K.S.; Liu, J.; Marina, O.; Napadow, V.; Haselgrove, C.; Kwong, K.K.; Kennedy, D.M.; Makris, N. The integrated response of the human cerebro-cerebellar and limbic systems to acupuncture stimulation at ST36 as evidenced by fMRI. *NeuroImage* **2005**, *27*, 479–496.

13. Dhond, R.P.; Yeh, C.; Park, K.; Kettner, N.; Napadow, V. Acupuncture modulates resting state connectivity in default and sensorimotor brain networks. *Pain* **2008**, *136*, 407–418.

14. Napadow, V.; Kettner, N.; Liu, J.; Li, M.; Kwong, K.K.; Vangel, M.; Makris, N.; Audette, J.; Hui, K.K. Hypothalamus and amygdala response to acupuncture stimuli in carpal tunnel syndrome. *Pain* **2007**, *130*, 254–266.

15. Wang, S.M.; Kain, Z.N.; White, P. Acupuncture Analgesia: I. The scientific basis. *Anesthesia Analgesia* **2008**, *106*, 602–610.

16. NIH consensus conference: Acupuncture. *JAMA* **1998**, *280*, 1518–1524. Wang, S.M.; Harris, R.E.; Lin, Y.C.; Gan, T.J. Acupuncture in 21st century anesthesia: Is there a needle in the haystack? *Anesthesia Analgesia* **2013**, *116*, 1356–1359.

17. Wang, S.M.; Kain, Z.N.; White, P. Acupuncture analgesia: II. Clinical considerations. *Anesthesia Analgesia* **2008**, *106*, 611–621.

18. Haake, M.; Muller, H.H.; Brittinger, C. German acupuncture trials (GERAC) for chronic low back pain. *Arch. Intern. Med.* **2007**, *167*, 1892–1898.

19. Langevin, H.M.; Wayne, P.M.; MacPherson, H.; Schnyer, R.; Milley, M.R.; Napadow, V.; Lao, L.; Park, J.; Harris, R.E.; Cohen, M. Paradoxes in acupuncture research: strategies for moving forward. *J. Evid. Based Complementary Altern. Med.* **2011**, doi:10.1155/2011/180805.

20. MacPherson, H.; Maschino, A.C.; Lewith, G.; Foster, N.E.; Witt, C.; Vickers, A.J. Characteristics of acupuncture treatment associated with outcome: An individual patient meta-analysis of 17,922 patients with chronic pain in randomized controlled trials. *PLoS ONE* **2013**, doi:10.1371/journal.pone.0077438.

21. Zeltzer, L.K.; Tsao, J.C.I.; Stelling, C.; Powers, M.; Waterhouse, M. A phase I study on the feasibility and acceptability of an acupuncture/hypnosis intervention for chronic pediatric pain. *J. Pain Symptom Manage.* **2002**, *24*, 437–446.

22. Lin, Y.; Bioteau, A.B.; Lee, A.C. Acupuncture for the management of pediatric pain. *Acupuncture Med.* **2003**, *14*, 45–46.

23. Kemper, K.J.; Sarah, R.; Silver-Highfield, E.; Xiarhos, E.; Barnes, L.; Berde, C. On pins and needles? Pediatric pain patients' experience with acupuncture *Pediatrics* **2000**, *105*, 941–947.

24. Gold, J.I.; Nicolau, C.D.; Belmont, K.A.; Katz, A.R.; Benaron, D.M.; Yu, W. *Pediatric Acupunct.* **2009**, *6*, 429–439.

25. Jastrowski Mano, K.E.; Davies, H. Parental attitudes toward acupuncture in a community sample. *J. Altern. Complement. Med.* **2009**, *15*, 661–668.

26. Meyer, R.M.L.; Barber, B.A.; Kobylecka, M.; Gold, J.I. Examining the association between parental stress related to child illness and child pain across acupuncture treatments. *Med. Acupunct.* **2014**, *26*, 23–30.

27. Adams, D.; Cheng, F.; Jou, H.; Aung, S.; Yasui, Y.; Vohra, S. The safety of pediatric acupuncture: A systematic review. *Pediatrics* **2011**; *128*, e1575–e1587.

28. Yates, C.C.; Mitchell, A.; Lowe, L.M.; Lee, A.; Hall, R.W. Safety of noninvasive electrical stimulation of acupuncture points during a routine neonatal heel stick. *Med. Acupunct.* **2013**, *25*, 285–290.

29. Allais, G.; de Lorenzo, C.; Quirico, P.; Airola, G.; Tolardo, G.; Mana, O.; Benedetto, C. Acupuncture in the prophylactic treatment of migraine without aura: a comparison with flumarizine. *Headache* **2002**, *42*, 855–861.

30. Diener, H.C.; Kronfeld, K.; Boewing, G.; Lungenhausen, M.; Maier, C.; Molsberger, A.; Tegenthoff, M.; Trampisch, H.J.; Zenz, M.; Meinert, R. Efficacy of acupuncture for the prophylaxis of migraine: a multicentre randomized controlled clinical trial. *Lancet Neurol.* **2006**, *5*, 310–316.

31. Linde, K.; Streng, A.; Hoppe, A.; Weidenhammer, W.; Wagenpfeil, S.; Melchart, D. Randomized trial *vs.* observational study of acupuncture for migraine found that patient characteristics differed but outcomes were similar. *J. Clin. Epidemiol.* **2007**, *60*, 280–287.

32. Linde, K.; Allais, G.; Brinkhaus, B.; Manheimer, E.; Vickers, A.; White, A.R. Acupuncture for migraine prophylaxis. *Cochrane Lib.* **2009**, doi:10.1002/14651858.CD001218.

33. Linde, K.; Allais, G.; Brinkhaus, B.; Manheimer, E.; Vickers, A.; White, A.R. Acupuncture for tension-type headache. *Cochrane Lib.* **2009**, doi:10.1002/14651858.CD007587.

34. Pintov, S.; Lahat, E.; Alstein, M.; Vogel, A.; Barg, J. Acupuncture and the opioid system: Implications in management of migraine. *Pediatr. Neurol.* **1997**, *17*, 129–133.

35. Gottschling, S.; Meyer, S.; Gribova, I.; Distler, L.; Berrang, J.; Gortner, L.; Graf, N.; Shamdeen, M.G. Laser acupuncture in children with headache: A double-blind, randomized, bicenter, placebo-controlled trial. *Pain* **2008**, *137*, 405–412.

36. Longstreth, G.F.; Thompson, W.G.; Chey, W.D.; Houghton, L.A.; Mearin, R.; Spiller, R.C. Functional bowel disorders. *Gastroenterology* **2006**, *130*, 1480–1491.

37. Chao, G.Q.; Zhang, S. Effectiveness of acupuncture to treat irritable bowel syndrome: A meta-analysis. *World J. Gastroenterol.* **2014**, *20*, 1871–1877.

38. Macpherson, H.; Tilbrook, H.; Bland, J.M.; Bloor, K.; Brabyn, S.; Cox, H.; Kang'ombe, A.R.; Man, M.S.; Stuardi, T.; Torgerson, D.; *et al.* Acupuncture for irritable bowel syndrome: primary care based pragmatic randomized controlled trial. *BMC Gastroenterol.* **2012**, *12*, 150.

39. Manheimer, E.; Cheng, K.; Wieland, L.S.; Min, L.S.; Shen, X.; Berman, B.H.; Lao, L. Acupuncture for treatment of irritable bowel syndrome. *Cochrane Lib.* **2012**, doi:10.1002/14651858.CD005111.pub3.review.

40. Hong, Y. The effects of hand-acupuncture therapy on intermittent abdominal pain in children. *Taehan Kanho Hakhoe Chi* **2005**, *35*, 487–93.

41. Buskila, D.; Ablin, J. Pediatric fibromyalgia. *Rheumatismo* **2012**, *64*, 230–237.

42. Anthony, K.K.; Shanberg, L.E. Juvenile primary fibromyalgia syndrome. *Curr. Rheumatology Rep.* **2001**, *3*, 165–171.

43. Tommaso, M.; Delussi, M.; Ricci, K.; D'Angelo, G. Abdominal acupuncture changes cortical responses to nociceptive stimuli in fibromyalgia patients. *CNS Neurosci. Ther.* **2014**, *20*, 565–567.

44. Cao, H.J.; Li, X.; Han, M.; Liu, J. Acupuncture stimulation for fibromyalgia: A systematic review of randomized controlled trials. *J. Evid. Based Complementary Altern. Med.* **2013**, doi:10.1155/2013/362831.

45. Tsao, J.C.I.; Meldrum, M.; Kim, S.C.; Jacob, M.C.; Zeltzer, L.K. Treatment preferences for CAM in Children with Chronic Pain. *Electron. Centralised Aircr. Monit.* **2007**, *4*, 367–374.

46. Toupin, A.K.; Walji, R. The state of research on complementary and alternative medicine in pediatric rheumatology. *Rheumatic Dis. Clin. N. Am.* **2011**, *37*, 85–94.

47. Hagen, L.E.; Schneider, R.; Stephens, D.; Modrusan, D.; Feldman, B.M. Use of complementary and alternative medicine by pediatric rheumatology patients. *Arthritis Rheumatol.* **2003**, *49*, 3–6.

48. April, K.T.; Ehrmann, F.D.; Zunzunegui, M.V.; Descarreaux, M.; Malleson, P.; Duffy, C.M. Longitudinal analysis of complementary and alternative health care use in children with juvenile idiopathic arthritis. *Complement. Ther. Med.* **2009**, *17*, 208–215.

49. Berman, B.M.; Lao, L.X.; Langenberg, P.; Lee, W.L.; Gilpin, A.M.; Hochberg, M.C. Effectiveness of acupuncture as adjunctive therapy in osteoarthritis of the knee. *Ann. Internal Med.* **2004**, *141*, 901–910.

50. Manheimer, E.; Linde, K.; Lao, L.X.; Bouter, L.M.; Berman, B.M. Meta-analysis: Acupuncture for osteoarthritis of the knee. *Ann. Internal Med.* **2007**, *146*, 868–877.

51. Zanette, S. de A.; Born, I.G.; Brenol, J.C.; Xavier, R.M. A pilot study of acupuncture as adjunctive treatment of rheumatoid arthritis. *Clin. Rheumatol.* **2008**, *27*, 627–635.

52. Kiran, G.; Gumusalan, Y.; Ekerbicer, H.C.; Kiran, H.; Coskun, A.; Arikan, D.C. A randomized pilot study of acupuncture treatment for primary dysmenorrhea. *Eur. J. Obstetrics Gynecology Reproductive Biol.* **2013**, *169*, 292–295.

53. Smith, C.A.; Zhu, X.; He, L.; Song, J. Acupuncture for primary dymenorrhoea. *Cochrane Rev.* **2011**, doi:10.1002/14651858.CD007854.pub2.

54. Yeh, M.L.; Hung, Y.L.; Chen, H.H.; Wang, Y.J. Auricular acupressure for pain relief in adolescents with dysmenorrhoea: A placebo controlled study. *J. Altern. Complement. Med.* **2013**, *19*, 313–318.

55. Wayne, P.M.; Kerr, C.E.; Schnyer, R.N.; Legedza, A.T.; Savetsky-German, J.; Shields, M.H.; Buring, J.E.; Davis, R.B.; Conboy, L.A.; Highfield, E. Japanese-style acupuncture for endometriosis-related pelvic pain in adolescents and young women: results of a randomized sham-controlled trial. *J. Pediatr. Adolescent Gynecol.* **2008**, *212*, 47–57.

56. Hommer, D.H. Chinese scalp acupuncture relieves pain and restores function in complex regional pain syndrome. *Mil. Med.* **2012**, *177*, 1231–1234.

57. Sprague, M.; Chang, J.C. Integrative approach focusing on acupuncture in the treatment of chronic complex regional pain syndrome. *J. Altern. Complement. Med.* **2011**, *17*, 67–70.

58. Leo, K.C. Use of electrical stimulation at acupuncture points for the treatment of reflex sympathetic dystrophy in a child: A case report. *J. Phys. Thermophys.* **1983**, *63*, 957–959.

59. Kelly, A. Treatment of reflex sympathetic dystrophy in 3 pediatric patients using 7 external dragons. *J. Med. Acup.* **2004**, *15*, 29–30.

60. Falk, S.; Dickenson, A.H. Pain and nociception: Mechanisms of cancer-induced bone pain. *J. Clin. Oncol.* **2014**, *32*, 1647–1654.

61. Gottschling, S.; Meyer, S.; Langler, A.; Scharifi, G.; Ebinger, F.; Gronwald, B. Differences in use of complementary and alternative medicine between children and adolescents with cancer in Germany: A population based survey. *Pediatr. Blood Cancer* **2014**, *61*, 488–492.

62. Gottschling, S.; Reindl, T.K.; Meyer, S.; Berrang, J.; Henze, G.; Graeber, S.; Ong, M.F.; Graf, N. Acupuncture to alleviate chemotherapy-induced nausea and vomiting in pediatric oncology—a randomized multicenter crossover pilot trial. *Klin. Padiatr.* **2008**, *220*, 365–370.

63. Ladas, E.J.; Rooney, D.; Taromina, K.; Ndao, D.H.; Kelly, K.M. The safety of acupuncture in children and adolescents with cancer therapy-related thrombocytopenia. *Supportive Care Cancer* **2010**, *18*, 1487–1490.

64. Wu, S.; Sapru, A.; Stewart, M.A.; Milet, M.J.; Hudes, M.; Livermore, L.F.; Flori, H.R. Using acupuncture for acute pain in hospitalized children. *Pediatr. Crit. Care Med.* **2009**, *10*, 291–296.

65. Lin, Y.C.; Tassone, R.F.; Jahng, S.; Rahbar, R.; Holzman, R.S.; Zurakowski, D.; Sethna, N. Acupuncture management of pain and emergence agitation in children after bilateral myringotomy and tympanostomy tube insertion. *Pediatr. Anesthesia* **2009**, *19*, 1096–1101.

66. Hollifield, M.; Sinclair-Lian, N.; Warner, T.D.; Hammerschlag, R. Acupuncture for posttraumatic stress disorder: A randomized controlled pilot trial. *J. Nerv. Mental Dis.* **2007**, *195*, 504–513.

67. Zhang, Y.; Feng, B.; Xie, J.P.; Xu, F.Z.; Chen, J. Clinical study on treatment of the earthquake-caused post-traumatic stress disorder by cognitive-behavior therapy and acupoint stimulation. *J. Trad. Chin. Med.* **2011**, *31*, 60–63.

68. Wang, S.M.; Escalera, S.; Lin, E.C.; Maranets, I.; Kain, Z.N. Extra-1 acupressure for children undergoing anesthesia. *Anesthesia Analgesia* **2008**, *107*, 811–816.

69. Kundu, A.; Jimenez, N.; Lynn, A. Acupuncture therapy for prevention of emergence delirium in children undergoing general anesthesia. *Med. Acupunct.* **2008**, *20*, 151–154.

70. Schwartz, L.; Xiao, R.; Brown, E.R.; Sommers, E. Auricular acupressure augmentation of standard medical management of the neonatal Narcotic Abstinence Syndrome. *Med. Acupunct.* **2011**, *23*, 175–186.

71. King, E.W.; Audette, K.; Athman, G.A.; Nguyen, H.O.; Sluka, K.A.; Fairbanks, C.A. Transcutaneous electrical nerve stimulation activates peripherally located alpha-2A adrenergic receptors. *Pain* **2005**, *115*, 364–373.

72. Wang, H.; Xie, Y.; Zhang, Q.; Xu, N.; Zhong, H.; Dong, H.; Liu, L.; Jiang, T.; Wang, Q.; Xiong, L. Transcutaneous electric acupoint stimulation reduced intra-operative remifentanil consumption and alleviates postoperative side-effects in patients undergoing sinusotomy: A prospective, randomized, placebo-controlled trial. *Br. J. Anaesthesia* **2014**, *112*, 1075–1082.

73. Kabalak, A.A.; Akcay, M.; Akcay, F.; Gogus, K. Transcutaneous electrical acupoint stimulation versus ondansetron in the prevention of postoperative vomiting following pediatric tonsillectomy. *J. Altern. Complement. Med.* **2005**, *11*, 407–413.

74. Ni, X.; Xie, Y.; Wang, Q.; Zhong, H.; Chen, M.; Wang, F.; Xiong, L. Cardioprotective effect of transcutaneous electric acupoint stimulation in the pediatric cardiac patients: a randomized controlled clinical trial. *Pediatr. Anesthesia* **2012**, *22*, 805–811.

75. Chi, H.; Zhou, W.X.; Wu, Y.Y.; Chen, T.Y.; Ge, W.; Yuan, L.; Shen, W.D.; Zhou, J. Electroacupuncture intervention combined with general anesthesia for 80 cases of heart valve replacement surgery under cardiopulmonary bypass. *Zhen Ci Yan Jiu* **2013**, *39*, 1–6.
76. Ferreira, D.C.; DeRossi, A.; Torres, C.P.; Galo, R.; Paula-Silva, F.W.; Queiroz, A.M. Effect of laser acupuncture and auricular acupressure in a child with trismus as a sequel of medulloblastoma. *Acupunct. Med.* **2013**, *32*, 190–193.
77. Thomas, K.H.; MacPherson, H.; Ratcliffe, J.; Thorpe, L.; Brazier, J.; Campbell, M.; Fitter, M.; Roman, M. Longer term clinical and economic benefits of offering acupuncture care to patients with chronic low back pain. *Health Technol. Assess.* **2005**, *9*, 1–109.

Integrative Treatment of Reflux and Functional Dyspepsia in Children

Ann Ming Yeh and Brenda Golianu

Abstract: Gastroesophageal reflux disease (GERD) and functional dyspepsia (FD) are common problems in the pediatric population, with up to 7% of school-age children and up to 8% of adolescents suffering from epigastric pain, heartburn, and regurgitation. Reflux is defined as the passage of stomach contents into the esophagus, while GERD refers to reflux symptoms that are associated with symptoms or complications—such as pain, asthma, aspiration pneumonia, or chronic cough. FD, as defined by the Rome III classification, is a persistent upper abdominal pain or discomfort, not related to bowel movements, and without any organic cause, that is present for at least two months prior to diagnosis. Endoscopic examination is typically negative in FD, whereas patients with GERD may have evidence of esophagitis or gastritis either grossly or microscopically. Up to 70% of children with dyspepsia exhibit delayed gastric emptying. Treatment of GERD and FD requires an integrative approach that may include pharmacologic therapy, treating concurrent constipation, botanicals, mind body techniques, improving sleep hygiene, increasing physical activity, and traditional Chinese medicine and acupuncture.

Reprinted from *Children*. Cite as: Yeh, A.M.; Golianu, B. Integrative Treatment of Reflux and Functional Dyspepsia in Children. *Children* **2014**, *1*, 119-133.

1. Introduction

Gastroesophageal reflux is the normal physiologic passage of gastric contents into the esophagus. When reflux and regurgitation cause symptoms and complications, it is defined as gastroesophageal reflux disease, or GERD. Symptoms of GERD include heartburn, epigastric pain, feeding difficulties, dysphagia, and aerodigestive symptoms such as asthma, chronic cough, or recurrent pneumonia. On upper endoscopy, GERD patients exhibit erosive esophagitis or gastritis. Functional dyspepsia (FD) is defined by the ROME III criteria as a persistent upper abdominal pain or discomfort that: (1) is not exclusively relieved by defecation or associated with the onset of a change in stool frequency or stool form; and (2) organic disease is unlikely to explain the symptoms. The pain or discomfort in the upper abdomen has to be present at least once per week for at least two months prior to diagnosis. Endoscopic examination is negative in FD both grossly and microscopically. Dyspepsia is reported in 5%–10% of otherwise healthy adolescents [1].

Treatment for GERD symptoms often includes an empiric trial of acid suppression. Histamine-2 receptor antagonists and proton pump inhibitors are often effective in healing esophagitis and treating symptoms of reflux. However, acid suppressing medications have significant side effects or long-term risks that may limit their use. Pharmacologic therapies with acid suppression do not always effectively treat symptoms related to non-erosive reflux disease and reflux symptoms from non-acidic reflux. Therefore, treatment of GERD and FD suggests an integrative medicine approach.

Integrative medicine is a healing oriented medicine that takes account of the whole patient, including all elements of lifestyle and family health. It emphasizes the powerful triad of patient-family-practitioner, is informed by evidence, and makes use of all appropriate therapies. In patients with GERD and FD, an integrative medicine treatment plan may include botanicals, mind-body techniques, sleep hygiene, increasing physical activity, and acupuncture, in addition to pharmacologic therapies. This paper will illustrate the integrative medicine approach with a case study and review the current scientific evidence on integrative medicine treatments for GERD and FD in children and adolescents.

2. Case Report

An 11-year old girl presented to outpatient gastroenterology clinic with abdominal pain and chronic nausea for the past month. Her abdominal pain was daily, 3–4/10 in intensity, and in the epigastric area. She described the nausea as occurring almost every hour on a daily basis. She had one episode of non-bloody, non-bilious vomiting while at summer camp, but since then has had only chronic nausea. She reported several days of school absence in the last month. Her primary pediatrician initially started famotidine, which partially improved pain but not nausea. She had been constipated for several months, and strained often to stool. She denied diarrhea, fever, tenesmus, hematochezia, or pain on defecation. She reported no weight loss, normal PO intake and appetite. She recently restricted dairy, and although this change did not improve her pain, she described episodes where she felt particularly nauseated after eating ice cream. For breakfast, she usually ate toast pops or cereal with fruit. Lunch was the typical school hot lunch with could include pizza, spaghetti, chicken nuggets, or a sandwich. Dinner was often eaten at home, and parents reported a healthy home-cooked organic diet that included meat.

Her past medical history was negative for surgeries, hospitalizations, or major infections. Her mother also has a history of constipation. She was in the 6th grade and with good grades, and had a sister in college. Parents both worked for a successful company they started together and endorsed increased work stress at home. She slept well from 9:30 pm to 6:30 am each night, was rested upon waking, but sometimes had trouble falling asleep. She described herself as a worrier and the caretaker of the family. Both mom and patient recognized that she could be sensitive, and she felt sad and worried when her parents were away. She described herself as easygoing with other kids in her class. Her main physical activity was during physical education class at school, and she did not exercise much otherwise.

On physical exam, her height is the 25th percentile, weight was at the 8th percentile, and BMI was at the 10th percentile. Abdominal exam was notable for hard stool palpable in the right ascending colon, and mild epigastric tenderness. Her physical exam was otherwise benign. Infectious stool studies for salmonella, shigella, campylobacter, Escherichia coli, giardia, cryptosporidium, and ova and parasites were all negative.

Her initial treatment plan included a trial of acid suppression with lansoprazole 30 mg a day for 4 weeks. She was also started on Miralax at 8.5 g–17 g/day to titrate to soft mushy stools and to increase fiber and fluids in her diet. She was advised to continue diary restriction and add a calcium supplement of 1000 mg a day. In addition, a trial of 0.5 mg of melatonin at bedtime was suggested to help with sleep latency. She was instructed to do moderate physical activity daily outside of PE class. Her nausea and epigastric pain did not improve with these initial measures, and she underwent upper endoscopy with biopsies. Endoscopy showed normal anatomy, mucosa and pathology and patient was subsequently given the diagnosis of functional dyspepsia.

Lansoprazole was discontinued given her lack of improvement, and parents were introduced to integrative treatment modalities. She started acupuncture treatments every other week along with a trial of gut-directed clinical hypnosis.

On traditional Chinese medicine (TCM) exam, her tongue exam revealed a tongue with a thin white coating that was dry appearing, scalloping at the lateral tongue edges and a puffy red and pink tip. Her pulse exam revealed a soft deep pulse at the third positions bilaterally, an empty pulse at the second position on the right, and wiry pulse at the second position on the left. This indicates potential TCM diagnosis of SP and KI Qi deficiency. Her acupuncture treatments consisted of Seirin J-type (0.16 × 30 mm) needles inserted at ST36 and LI4 points bilaterally. Alcohol prep was used on the skin prior to insertion of needles. Pointer Plus ear point finder was used to find reactive auricular acupuncture points and gold beads were placed at the ear points "esophagus", "spleen", and "liver" on one ear, alternating sides at the following visit. Body magnets were placed at SP9, SP6, PC6, TH5, and ST43 bilaterally. Patient was instructed to remove magnets and beads in 3 days unless they fell off sooner. In addition, she was instructed to apply additional magnets on points PC6 and ST43 on an as needed basis at home. These acupuncture and acupressure points were chosen to treat constipation, to clear inflammation, and to tonify SP and KI Qi. Points PC6 and ST43 in particular were chosen to treat nausea. At our institution, nausea and dyspepsia are commonly treated with the points listed above; a standard combination includes PC6 and ST43 (nausea), LI 4 and ST 36 (if constipation plays a role), SP6 and SP9 (SP qi deficiency), and CV 10 and 12 (dyspepsia). The choice of acupuncture *versus* acupressure and exact combination of points depends on patient tolerance and the patient's overall constellation of symptoms. This patient specifically did not desire any abdominal points, and therefore CV10 and CV12 were avoided.

Her gut-directed clinical hypnosis sessions were particularly helpful, and she was able to record the sessions on her tablet computer and use them as needed at home. During her hypnosis sessions with her trained therapist, she revealed that family discord and stress from her parents significantly worsened her symptoms. Parents received counseling from the therapist and tried to avoid stressful conversations in front of the patient. She was also started on ginger chews, ginger tea, and deglycyrrhizinated licorice on an as needed basis for nausea. Physical activity was encouraged, and she reported that walking after meals helped relieve postprandial fullness.

After a course of acupuncture, hypnotherapy, and the above interventions, she felt significant improvement in symptoms, with minimal nausea, excellent weight gain, and no further school absences. When she did feel more nauseated, she would self-apply acupressure magnets or listen to pre-recorded clinical hypnosis sessions as needed.

3. Treatment of GERD and Dyspepsia

3.1. Pharmacologic

Medications for GERD include histamine-2 receptor antagonists, proton pump inhibitors, and mucosal surface barriers and gastric acid buffering agents. Prokinetics are less frequently used.

First line medications include histamine-2 receptor antagonists (H2RA's) such as ranitidine, cimetidine, famotidine, and nitazidine. The histamine-2 receptors are found on the acid producing parietal cells of the stomach mucosa, and blockage of these receptors partially decreases production of stomach acid, typically within 30 min of administration, with the effect lasting for 6 h [2]. Tachyphylaxis, or a tolerance to the medication and a decreased treatment response, occurs after several weeks and thereby may limit long-term use [3].

Proton pump inhibitors (PPI's) such as omeprazole, esomeprazole, and lansoprazole are second line agents for increased acid suppression. These medications block acid secretion by inhibition of the sodium-potassium-ATPase pump. PPI's are superior to H2RA's in acid suppression and for erosive esophagitis. The efficacy of PPI's also does not decrease with long-term use, as compared to H2RA's. In older children and adolescents, a patient with classic GERD symptoms may warrant an empiric trial of acid suppression to determine if symptoms are related to acid reflux. In an older child or adolescent with symptoms suggestive of GERD, The North American Society of Pediatric Gastroenterology and Nutrition (NASPGAN) clinical guidelines recommend an empiric 4 week trial of a proton pump inhibitor (PPI) to determine if symptoms respond [4]. However, treatment response does not confirm a GERD diagnosis because it may reflect a spontaneous resolution of symptoms or a placebo. Upper endoscopy may be recommended to confirm diagnosis if patient does not respond to empiric acid blockade or if unable to wean off medication.

The most common reported side effects of acid suppressing medications include constipation, headache, nausea, and diarrhea, which occur with an incidence of 2%–7% [4]. Gastric acid serves as a part of the body's innate immune system. Reviews of the pediatric literature also raise concerns for an increased incidence of infections in patients exposed to acid suppression [5]. Previously healthy pediatric patients diagnosed with GERD and treated with either ranitidine or omeprazole had a higher incidence of pneumonia (12% *vs.* 2%, $p < 0.05$) and acute gastroenteritis (42% *vs.* 20% $p = 0.001$) during the 4 month follow up compared to healthy controls [6]. Adult studies also associate long-term PPI use with increased risk of nutrient malabsorption for calcium, iron, magnesium and vitamin B12. Because of decreased calcium or B12 absorption, an increased fall and fracture risk is also reported in the elderly population after long-term (>1 year) PPI use [7,8]. Furthermore, after PPI treatment in healthy volunteers for 8 weeks, PPI's induced acid related withdrawal symptoms secondary to rebound acid hypersecretion [9]. Patients often report difficulty weaning off PPI's secondary to rebound symptoms.

There is little evidence to justify the treatment of GERD and dyspepsia with promotility agents such as cisapride, erythromycin and metoclopramide. Although effective at increasing gastric motility and decreasing reflux symptoms, cisapride, a serotonin receptor agonist, was withdrawn from the market in the United States due to complications with fatal arrhythmias, long QT syndrome, and sudden death. Erythromycin, an antibiotic, also has promotility effects when administered at low doses

(1–3 mg/kg) to stimulate gastric antral motility. However, the studies are limited to patients with delayed gastric emptying and dysmotility, and to date there is insufficient evidence for treating GERD and dyspepsia [4,10]. Metoclopromide is also a dopamine antagonist that has been shown to decrease reflux index and daily symptoms [11]. However, given the potential for extrapyramidal side effects, including irreversible tardive dyskinesia, the side effect profile of metoclopromide greatly limits its use in clinical practice [12,13].

Antacids buffer gastric acid contents, and decrease reflux symptoms and can aid in healing erosive esophagitis. However, formal studies using pH or impedance monitoring have not been performed in children. Mucosal surface protective agents with alginate or sucralfate also have limited evidence in pediatrics, though sucralfate may be as effective as cimetidine for healing erosive esophagitis. Long-term sucralfate use should be used with caution due to unknown risk of aluminum toxicity in children.

3.2. Diet

Patients with reflux often benefit from a diet that avoids specific food triggers. In particular, fatty foods, spicy foods, acidic foods, chocolate, and caffeine worsen reflux symptoms. Some patients with food sensitivities or an allergic component to their symptoms may benefit from an elimination diet. Elimination diets systematically remove and then reintroduce common allergic triggers such as dairy, wheat, egg, nuts, or fish to look for symptom improvement upon elimination and symptom worsening upon reintroduction. Prior to completely eliminating wheat, a celiac screen should be performed with a tissue transglutaminase IgA antibody, and a total IgA level.

3.3. Other Motility Concerns: Constipation

Constipation and fecal retention can worsen GERD and dyspepsia symptoms in all age groups, and constipation and reflux often co-exist. In a study of children aged 4–16 years old with functional constipation diagnosed by Rome III criteria, approximately 40% of these patients presented with pathologic acid reflux by 24 h esophageal pH monitoring [14]. Constipation can also significantly affect overall GI motility. Rectal distension impaired gastric slow waves in healthy volunteers [15]. An association with reflux symptoms and constipation may be particularly prominent in children with underlying neurologic problems, underlying motility problems, or in patients with dysmotility after infectious enteritis [16]. Therefore, treating concurrent constipation with diet or laxatives can improve reflux symptoms.

3.4. Botanicals and Supplements

Various botanicals have been studied in the treatment of GERD and functional dyspepsia. Although studies on herbal remedies are small and with varied results, certain botanicals such as Iberogast (STW-5), deglycyrrhizinated licorice, and ginger show good potential for treating reflux symptoms with few adverse effects. Patients with severe reflux should be cautioned against using non-enteric coated peppermint, as it has been shown to relax the lower esophageal sphincter and potentially worsen reflux symptoms [17].

3.4.1. Iberogast

Iberogast (STW-5—Medical Futures Inc., Richmond Hill, Ontario, Canada) is a commercial preparation of 9 herbal extracts including bitter candy tuft, lemon balm leaf, chamomile flower, caraway fruit, licorice root, angelica root, milk thistle fruit, peppermint leaf, and greater celandine herb. In vitro, it has been shown to protect against the development of ulcers with decreased acid production, increased mucin production, an increase in prostaglandin E2 release, and a decrease in leukotrienes [18]. Although the evidence is mixed, clinical studies suggest that it acts directly to increase gastric motility in healthy subjects by increasing the motility index of antral pressure waves [19], but not necessarily decrease the overall gastric emptying time [20]. A review of the 12 clinical studies on Iberogast concluded that it is both safe and effective for treatment of functional dyspepsia and irritable bowel syndrome. The incidence of adverse drug reactions in this review was reported to be 0.04% and was mainly in the form of hypersensitivity reactions such as skin irritation, dyspnea, and pruritis [21]. The low incidence of adverse events and excellent safety profile is confirmed by the spontaneous reporting system in Germany and worldwide since the product was introduced approximately 50 years ago. Although no studies on efficacy exist in children, the preliminary adult studies and excellent safety profile are encouraging.

3.4.2. Licorice

Licorice root, the dried rhizome or extracts of *glycyrrhiza glabra*, has long been used in botanical medicine for treatment of gastric inflammation. The mechanism of action is thought to be due to inhibition of prostaglandin synthesis and lipoxygenase [22]. Glycyrrhizin has mineralocorticoid properties, and therefore the deglycyrrhizinated form of licorice is recommended for long-term or higher doses. Deglycyrrhizinated licorice (DGL) and licorice extracts without the glycyrrhizin do not have side effects of hyperkalemia, hypertension, and sodium retention [22]. In a small, randomized, double-blind, placebo controlled study of 50 adults with functional dyspepsia as diagnosed by Rome III criteria, subjects were randomized to placebo or a 75 mg extract of *Glycyrrhiza glabra* (GutGard®, Karnataka, India) for 30 days. Symptoms were assessed with a 7-point Likert scale of dyspepsia symptom severity at day 0, 15, and 30. Compared to placebo, the licorice extract showed a significant decrease in total symptom scores ($p < 0.05$) and improvement in quality of life [23]. Although more evidence is needed, integrative medicine practitioners frequently use deglycyrrhizinated licorice to help wean off acid suppression.

3.4.3. Ginger

Ginger root, the rhizome of *Zingiber officinale*, has been used traditionally as a kitchen spice but also for treating reflux symptoms and dyspepsia. Adult studies have demonstrated efficacy of ginger to treat pregnancy-induced nausea and vomiting, postoperative nausea, and drug induced nausea and vomiting [24–28]. Ginger root has a prokinetic effect that may be mediated by cholinergic action and spasmogenic properties that have been demonstrated in mouse and guinea pig models [29,30]. In healthy volunteers, both Wu [31] and Micklefield [32] showed ginger root improved gastric emptying and gastroduodenal motility in both the fasting and fed state. The recommended dose ranges from 1 g to 1.5 g of the dried herb per day, with administration typically 30 min to 1 h before a meal. It is important to note the ginger rhizome extract is much more concentrated than the dried ginger root powder. When used in typical doses, most patients tolerate ginger well. Side effects are reported when doses exceed 5 g/day and include heartburn, abdominal discomfort and diarrhea. Ginger root has been shown to have an antiplatelet effect due to its ability to inhibit platelet thromboxane [33]. Therefore, it is relatively contraindicated in patients with a bleeding disorder, and should be discontinued prior to surgical procedures.

In terms of safety in pediatrics, no trials to date have investigated ginger and safety in children; though the use of ginger in pregnant women is likely safe with no increased risk of congenital malformations or harm to the fetus. In children who are unable to swallow ginger root capsules, ginger candies, chews and teas are often more palatable.

3.4.4. Peppermint

Although there is some evidence that enteric coated peppermint oil may be effective in treating irritable bowel syndrome in adults and in children [34,35], caution should be used for peppermint oil in patients with reflux. Peppermint is known to have anti-spasmodic activity on smooth muscles, and may increase relaxation of the lower esophageal sphincter. This could exacerbate reflux symptoms, especially in patients with erosive esophagitis or hiatal hernia [17].

3.5. Sleep Hygiene and Melatonin

Melatonin is a naturally occurring hormone produced by the pineal gland in the brain. It is produced with the onset of darkness and inhibited by exposure to light on the retina. It regulates the sleep-wake cycle and serves as a darkness signal but is not sedating. Melatonin levels are low in the daytime. Endogenous production rises at night and peaks between 11 pm and 3 am [36].

In addition to its effects on the sleep-wake cycle, emerging evidence suggests that melatonin also has a gastroprotective effect. Melatonin production by the enterochromaffin cells in the digestive mucosa exceeds pineal gland production after tryptophan stimulation [37,38]. Melatonin in the GI tract has been shown *in vitro* to regulate GI motility, modulate visceral sensation, and produce an anti-inflammatory response [39].

A study by Klupinska *et al.* [40] found that patients with GERD and recurrent peptic ulcer disease had decreased levels of nighttime peak melatonin compared to those with non-erosive reflux disease and functional dyspepsia, suggesting a protective effect of melatonin on the upper GI mucosa. A small randomized controlled trial of 27 adults with GERD found that 3 mg of melatonin alone at bedtime was effective in treating GERD symptoms over placebo [41]. Another small trial by Kandil *et al.* [41] randomized GERD patients into 4 treatment groups: placebo, 3 mg of immediate release melatonin, 20 mg of omeprazole, or melatonin plus omeprazole for 8 weeks. Although omeprazole alone was more effective at symptom improvement than melatonin alone, melatonin alone was more effective than placebo. Furthermore, the addition of melatonin to omeprazole provided a synergistic effect and increased the efficacy of omeprazole. Interestingly, patients in both melatonin groups had significantly higher LES sphincter pressures on manometry compared to both the omeprazole only group and controls. Another head-to-head trial compared 20 mg of omeprazole to a supplement containing melatonin (6 mg), its precursor L-tryptophan (200 mg), B vitamins and folic acid for 40 days in 350 patients with GERD. 100% of patients in the supplement group had regression of symptoms, compared to 66% of the omeprazole group [42]. All studies reported no significant side effects or complications of melatonin supplementation. Although these adult studies are small and need further replication, they suggest a significant gastroprotective effect of both endogenous and exogenous melatonin.

In children with delayed sleep phase disorder and prolonged sleep latency, short-term supplementation of melatonin at low doses in children is generally regarded as safe and well tolerated [43–45]. Side effects include early morning grogginess, somnolence, dizziness and headaches. Effective dosing in children ranges from 0.3 mg to 5 mg, and oftentimes doses of 0.3 mg to 1 mg are sufficient to improve sleep latency. Further research is needed to investigate the role of melatonin and efficacy on the GI tract diseases in children.

Sleep disruptions can significantly decrease normal melatonin production and thereby affect the gastroprotective effect on the mucosal lining. Poor sleep quality is associated with increased acid exposure, increased exacerbations of reflux the following day, and visceral hyperalgesia [46,47]. Working to improving the child's sleep hygiene may help increase the physiologic production of melatonin and decrease visceral hypersensitivity. Important elements of a sleep history include sleep quality, sleep latency (time it takes to transition from full wakefulness to sleep), night waking, daytime drowsiness, and exposure to light at night. Improving a patient's sleep hygiene includes eliminating use of electronics one hour prior to bedtime, earlier bedtime, and improving the overall quality of sleep.

3.6. Acupuncture and Acupressure

Acupuncture, a healing modality used in traditional Chinese medicine, uses fine needles inserted at defined acupuncture points to balance the body's Qi, or life energy. In traditional Chinese medicine, a patient is evaluated for imbalances or blockages in the body's Qi, and acupuncture is employed as part of a holistic treatment approach. Treatments may include Chinese herbs, massage, and movement-based therapies such as Tai Qi or QiGong. Specifically for reflux and dyspepsia, certain acupuncture points such as PC6 (*neiguan*), and ST36 (*zusanli*) have been effective in improving reflux symptoms, nausea, and vomiting. Research on these two points has also started to pinpoint the physiologic mechanism of action.

PC6 (*neiguan*), on the pericardium meridian, is one of the most used and investigated acupuncture points for nausea, vomiting, and reflux. The point is located in the groove caudal to the flexor carpi radialis and cranial to the superficial digital flexor muscles. Acupuncture and electrical stimulation of PC6 has been shown to be as effective as antiemetics in adults with nausea and vomiting induced by chemotherapy, pregnancy, and postoperative settings [48–50]. In children, both auricular acupuncture and body acupuncture have improved postoperative and chemotherapy induced nausea and vomiting [51–54]. Furthermore, functional MRI studies have shown increased attenuation of the cerebrocerebellum after acupuncture on point PC6 over control points, suggesting modulation of cerebellar activities [55].

ST36 (*zusanli*), on the stomach meridian, is located at the proximal one-fifth of the craniolateral surface of the rear leg, distal to the head of the tibia in a depression between the muscles of the cranial tibia and the extensor digitalis longus. In healthy men, electrical acupuncture at ST36 decreases basal acid output and gastric acid secretion, increases pancreatic polypeptide levels, and increases amplitude of gastric antral contractions [56].

Other acupuncture points that have been traditionally used for GERD and dyspepsia include the following points, especially if found to be tender to touch: ST43 (*xiangu*), CV12 (*zhongwan*), ST25 (*tianshu*), SP4 (*gongsun*), LV3 (*taicong*), BL21 (*weishu*), and LI4 (*hegu*). The above points may also be used in combinations in a clinical treatment, as indicated by the presenting complaint and Chinese medical pattern diagnosis. However, these individual points have not been studied extensively in clinical studies, and further research is required to evaluate efficacy.

There are no published clinical trials to date on acupuncture and acupressure in children with reflux or dyspepsia. However, the safety of acupuncture in children is well documented. One review of the literature cites a 1.55 risk of any adverse events occurring in 100 treatments of acupuncture [57]. Puncture redness is the most commonly reported side effect, followed by needle pain, and light-headedness. A serious adverse event is defined as an event that is life threatening or requires hospitalization. Studies have reported this risk to be as low as 0.05/10,000 treatments in the general population [57]. In addition to acupuncture, non-invasive forms of acupressure are available for pediatrics using laser acupuncture, topical magnets, and acupressure beads. These may be preferred by needle phobic children or in high-risk patients who may be immunosuppressed or at a risk for bleeding. They may also be used as adjunctive treatments following needle placement.

3.7. Mind Body Therapy

Psychosocial stressors may exacerbate symptoms in many children with GERD and FD. Compared with healthy controls, FD patients are more likely to exhibit psychological distress, somatization, anxiety and depression [58]. Adult patients with dyspepsia also have a higher reported incidence of childhood emotional abuse [59]. It is therefore important to address the mind-body-gut connection when treating a patient with GERD or FD. Patients with significant anxiety and depression may benefit from psychiatric evaluation or counseling. All children with increased psychosocial stressors and mild anxiety can benefit from mind-body therapies and relaxation techniques. Types of mind-body therapy include mindfulness meditation, guided imagery, biofeedback, clinical hypnosis, and yoga. Treatment can be tailored to the interest and motivation of the individual patient.

Gut directed hypnotherapy is a form of clinical hypnosis that is based on muscular and mental relaxation. General hypnotic suggestions are used to either focus on the symptoms or to distract from them. A Cochrane review in 2007 found hypnotherapy to be effective for irritable bowel syndrome in adults [60]. Hypnotherapy was effective in providing long-term symptom improvement and decreased medication use and consultation [61]. A small study of gut-directed hypnotherapy was found to shorten gastric emptying both in dyspeptic and in healthy subjects as measured by ultrasonography [62]. In children with functional abdominal pain or irritable bowel syndrome, three randomized control trials have been published to date. Van Tilburg *et al.* [63]

established that a home-based audio of guided imagery recordings using hypnotherapy techniques was more effective than standard care to improve pain symptoms in children with functional abdominal pain (63% *vs*. 27%). Studies by Weydert [64] and Vlieger [65] also demonstrated that gut directed hypnosis by a trained therapist was superior to standard care in pediatric patients with irritable bowel syndrome. Although all three of the above studies had small sample sizes (ranging from 22 to 52 patients), the efficacy results and excellent safety profile suggest that it is a likely beneficial treatment modality [66].

3.8. Obesity and Weight Loss

Obesity may predispose a patient to increased intragastric pressure, more frequent transient lower esophageal sphincter relaxations, and increased esophageal acid exposure. Although data is scarce in the pediatric population, adult studies have shown obesity to be correlated with increased incidence of GERD, Barrett's esophagus, and esophageal adenocarcinoma [67,68]. Jacobson's study of women with GERD symptoms showed that even moderate weight gain in person of normal weight caused or exacerbated reflux symptoms. A large prospective population-based cohort study further indicates that weight loss in patients with GER symptoms was dose-dependently associated with a symptom reduction. Weight loss was also associated with increased treatment success with antireflux medication [69]. Recommending weight loss or weight maintenance in obese and overweight children, and encouraging moderate physical activity in all children with GERD and FD should be an integral component to the treatment plan.

4. Conclusions

As illustrated by the case report and review of literature, patients with GERD and FD can benefit significantly from an integrative treatment approach. Pharmacologic medications such as H2-blockers and PPI's are effective at treating symptoms. However, side effects, long-term risks, and difficulty with discontinuation can limit their use. Botanicals such as Iberogast, DGL, and ginger can often provide adjunct symptomatic relief with a good safety profile. Emerging evidence suggests good sleep hygiene and melatonin secretion may play an important gastroprotective role in the GI tract. Furthermore, working with mind-body therapies and acupuncture may improve GERD symptoms, motility, and help with stress reduction. We encourage all pediatricians and pediatric gastroenterologists to consider an integrative and holistic approach when treating a patient with gastroesophageal reflux and functional dyspepsia.

Acknowledgements

The authors would like to thank The Stephen Bechtel Endowed Postdoctoral Fellowship as well as the Stanford CTSA (grant number UL1 RR025744) for contributing to the funding of this research.

Author Contributions

A.Y. and B.G. wrote the manuscript and commented on the manuscript at all stages.

Conflicts of Interest

The authors declare no conflict of interest.

References

1. Hyams, J.S.; Burke, G.; Davis, P.M.; Rzepski, B.; Andrulonis, P.A. Abdominal pain and irritable bowel syndrome in adolescents: A community-based study. *J. Pediatr.* **1996**, *129*, 220–226.
2. Orenstein, S.R.; Blumer, J.L.; Faessel, H.M.; McGuire, J.A.; Fung, K.; Li, B.U.; Lavine, J.E.; Grunow, J.E.; Treem, W.R.; Ciociola, A.A. Ranitidine, 75 mg, over-the-counter dose: Pharmacokinetic and pharmacodynamic effects in children with symptoms of gastro-oesophageal reflux. *Aliment. Pharmacol. Ther.* **2002**, *16*, 899–907.
3. Nwokolo, C.U.; Smith, J.T.; Gavey, C.; Sawyerr, A.; Pounder, R.E. Tolerance during 29 days of conventional dosing with cimetidine, nizatidine, famotidine or ranitidine. *Aliment. Pharmacol. Ther.* **1990**, *4*, S29–S45.
4. Vandenplas, Y.; Rudolph, C.D.; di Lorenzo, C.; Hassall, E.; Liptak, G.; Mazur, L.; Sondheimer, J.; Staiano, A.; Thomson, M.; Veereman-Wauters, G.; *et al.* Pediatric gastroesophageal reflux clinical practice guidelines: Joint recommendations of the North American Society for Pediatric Gastroenterology, Hepatology, and Nutrition (NASPGHAN) and the European Society for Pediatric Gastroenterology, Hepatology, and Nutrition (ESPGHAN). *J. Pediatr. Gastroenterol. Nutr.* **2009**, *49*, 498–547.
5. Chung, E.Y.; Yardley, J. Are there risks associated with empiric acid suppression treatment of infants and children suspected of having gastroesophageal reflux disease? *Hosp. Pediatr.* **2013**, *3*, 16–23.
6. Canani, R.B.; Cirillo, P.; Roggero, P.; Romano, C.; Malamisura, B.; Terrin, G.; Passariello, A.; Manguso, F.; Morelli, L.; Guarino, A.; *et al.* Therapy with gastric acidity inhibitors increases the risk of acute gastroenteritis and community-acquired pneumonia in children. *Pediatrics* **2006**, *117*, e817–e820.
7. Lewis, J.R.; Barre, D.; Zhu, K.; Ivey, K.L.; Lim, E.M.; Hughes, J.; Prince, R.L. Long-term proton pump inhibitor therapy and falls and fractures in elderly women: A prospective cohort study. *J. Bone Miner. Res.* **2014**, doi:10.1002/jbmr.2279.
8. Ding, J.; Heller, D.A.; Ahern, F.M.; Brown, T.V. The relationship between proton pump inhibitor adherence and fracture risk in the elderly. *Calcif. Tissue Int.* **2014**, *94*, 597–607.
9. Reimer, C.; Søndergaard, B.; Hilsted, L.; Bytzer, P. Proton-pump inhibitor therapy induces acid-related symptoms in healthy volunteers after withdrawal of therapy. *Gastroenterology* **2009**, *137*, 80–87.
10. Curry, J.I.; Lander, T.D.; Stringer, M.D. Review article: Erythromycin as a prokinetic agent in infants and children. *Aliment. Pharmacol. Ther.* **2001**, *15*, 595–603.

124

11. Craig, W.R.; Hanlon-Dearman, A.; Sinclair, C.; Taback, S.; Moffatt, M. Metoclopramide, thickened feedings, and positioning for gastro-oesophageal reflux in children under two years. *Cochrane Database Syst. Rev.* **2004**, doi:10.1002/14651858.CD003502.pub2.

12. Ganzini, L.; Casey, D.E.; Hoffman, W.F.; McCall, A.L. The prevalence of metoclopramide-induced tardive dyskinesia and acute extrapyramidal movement disorders. *Arch. Int. Med.* **1993**, *153*, 1469–1475.

13. Putnam, P.E.; Orenstein, S.R.; Wessel, H.B.; Stowe, R.M. Tardive dyskinesia associated with use of metoclopramide in a child. *J. Pediatr.* **1992**, *121*, 983–985.

14. Baran, M.; Özgenç, F.; Arikan, Ç.; Çakir, M.; Ecevıt, Ç.Ö.; Aydoğdu, S.; Yağci, R.V. Gastroesophageal reflux in children with functional constipation. *Turk. J. Gastroenterol.* **2012**, *23*, 634–638.

15. Liu, J.; Huang, H.; Xu, X.; Chen, J.D.Z. Effects and possible mechanisms of acupuncture at ST36 on upper and lower abdominal symptoms induced by rectal distension in healthy volunteers. *AJP Regul. Integr. Comp. Physiol.* **2012**, *303*, R209–R217.

16. Porter, C.K.; Faix, D.J.; Shiau, D.; Espiritu, J.; Espinosa, B.J.; Riddle, M.S. Postinfectious gastrointestinal disorders following norovirus outbreaks. *Clin. Infect. Dis.* **2012**, *55*, 915–922.

17. McKay, D.L.; Blumberg, J.B. A review of the bioactivity and potential health benefits of peppermint tea (*Mentha piperita* L.). *Phytother. Res. PTR* **2006**, *20*, 619–633.

18. Khayyal, M.T.; Seif-El-Nasr, M.; El-Ghazaly, M.A.; Okpanyi, S.N.; Kelber, O.; Weiser, D. Mechanisms involved in the gastro-protective effect of STW 5 (Iberogast) and its components against ulcers and rebound acidity. *Phytomed. Int. J. Phytother. Phytopharm.* **2006**, *13*, S56–S66.

19. Pilichiewicz, A.N.; Horowitz, M.; Russo, A.; Maddox, A.F.; Jones, K.L.; Schemann, M.; Holtmann, G.; Feinle-Bisset, C. Effects of Iberogast on proximal gastric volume, antropyloroduodenal motility and gastric emptying in healthy men. *Am. J. Gastroenterol.* **2007**, *102*, 1276–1283.

20. Braden, B.; Caspary, W.; Börner, N.; Vinson, B.; Schneider, A.R.J. Clinical effects of STW 5 (Iberogast) are not based on acceleration of gastric emptying in patients with functional dyspepsia and gastroparesis. *Neurogastroenterol. Motil.* **2009**, *21*, 632–638.

21. Ottillinger, B.; Storr, M.; Malfertheiner, P.; Allescher, H.-D. STW 5 (Iberogast®)—A safe and effective standard in the treatment of functional gastrointestinal disorders. *Wien. Med. Wochenschr.* **2013**, *163*, 65–72.

22. Schulz, V. *Rational Phytotherapy a Reference Guide for Physicians and Pharmacists*, 5th ed., fully rev. and expande; Springer: Berlin, Germany/New York, NY, USA, 2004.

23. Raveendra, K.R.; Jayachandra; Srinivasa, V.; Sushma, K.R.; Allan, J.J.; Goudar, K.S.; Shivaprasad, H.N.; Venkateshwarlu, K.; Geetharani, P.; Sushma, G.; *et al.* An extract of glycyrrhiza glabra (gutgard) alleviates symptoms of functional dyspepsia: A randomized, double-blind, placebo-controlled study. *Evid. Based Complement Alternat. Med.* **2012**, *2012*, 1–9.

24. Dabaghzadeh, F.; Khalili, H.; Dashti-Khavidaki, S. Ginger for prevention or treatment of drug-induced nausea and vomiting. *Curr. Clin. Pharmacol.* **2013**, PMID: 24218997.

25. Haji Seid Javadi, E.; Salehi, F.; Mashrabi, O. Comparing the effectiveness of vitamin b6 and ginger in treatment of pregnancy-induced nausea and vomiting. *Obstet. Gynecol. Int.* **2013**, *2013*, 927834.

26. Haniadka, R.; Saldanha, E.; Sunita, V.; Palatty, P.L.; Fayad, R.; Baliga, M.S. A review of the gastroprotective effects of ginger (*Zingiber officinale* Roscoe). *Food Funct.* **2013**, *4*, 845–855.

27. Marx, W.; McCarthy, A.L.; Ried, K.; Vitetta, L.; McKavanagh, D.; Thomson, D.; Sali, A.; Isenring, L. Can ginger ameliorate chemotherapy-induced nausea? Protocol of a randomized double blind, placebo-controlled trial. *BMC Complement. Altern. Med.* **2014**, *14*, 134.

28. Thomson, M.; Corbin, R.; Leung, L. Effects of ginger for nausea and vomiting in early pregnancy: A meta-analysis. *J. Am. Board Fam. Med. JABFM* **2014**, *27*, 115–122.

29. Ghayur, M.N.; Gilani, A.H. Pharmacological basis for the medicinal use of ginger in gastrointestinal disorders. *Dig. Dis. Sci.* **2005**, *50*, 1889–1897.

30. Ghayur, M.N.; Gilani, A.H. Species differences in the prokinetic effects of ginger. *Int. J. Food Sci. Nutr.* **2006**, *57*, 65–73.

31. Wu, K.-L.; Rayner, C.K.; Chuah, S.-K.; Changchien, C.S.; Lu, S.N.; Chiu, Y.C.; Chiu, K.W.; Lee, C.M. Effects of ginger on gastric emptying and motility in healthy humans. *Eur. J. Gastroenterol. Hepatol.* **2008**, *20*, 436–440.

32. Micklefield, G.H.; Redeker, Y.; Meister, V.; Jung, O.; Greving, I.; May, B. Effects of ginger on gastroduodenal motility. *Int. J. Clin. Pharmacol. Ther.* **1999**, *37*, 341–346.

33. Thomson, M.; Al-Qattan, K.K.; Al-Sawan, S.M.; Alnaqeeb, M.A.; Khan, I.; Ali, M. The use of ginger (*Zingiber officinale* Rosc.) as a potential anti-inflammatory and antithrombotic agent. *Prostaglandins Leukot Essent Fatty Acids.* **2002**, *67*, 475–478.

34. Leicester, R.J.; Hunt, R.H. Peppermint oil to reduce colonic spasm during endoscopy. *Lancet* **1982**, *2*, 989.

35. Kline, R.M.; Kline, J.J.; di Palma, J.; Barbero, G.J. Enteric-coated, pH-dependent peppermint oil capsules for the treatment of irritable bowel syndrome in children. *J. Pediatr.* **2001**, *138*, 125–128.

36. Zisapel, N. Sleep and sleep disturbances: Biological basis and clinical implications. *Cell Mol. Life Sci. CMLS* **2007**, *64*, 1174–1186.

37. Konturek, S.J.; Konturek, P.C.; Brzozowski, T.; Bubenik, G.A. Role of melatonin in upper gastrointestinal tract. *J. Physiol. Pharmacol.* **2007**, *58*, S23–S52.

38. Brzozowska, I.; Strzalka, M.; Drozdowicz, D.; Konturek, S.J.; Brzozowski, T. Mechanisms of esophageal protection, gastroprotection and ulcer healing by melatonin. implications for the therapeutic use of melatonin in Gastroesophageal Reflux Disease (GERD) and peptic ulcer disease. *Curr. Pharm. Des.* **2013**, PMID: 24251671.

39. Siah, K.T.H.; Wong, R.K.M.; Ho, K.Y. Melatonin for the treatment of irritable bowel syndrome. *World J. Gastroenterol.* **2014**, *20*, 2492–2498.

40. Klupińska, G.; Wiśniewska-Jarosińska, M.; Harasiuk, A.; Chojnacki, C.; Stec-Michalska, K.; Błasiak, J.; Reiter, R.J.; Chojnacki, J. Nocturnal secretion of melatonin in patients with upper digestive tract disorders. *J. Physiol. Pharmacol.* **2006**, *57*, S41–S50.

41. Kandil, T.S.; Mousa, A.A.; El-Gendy, A.A.; Abbas, A.M. The potential therapeutic effect of melatonin in Gastro-Esophageal Reflux Disease. *BMC Gastroenterol.* **2010**, *10*, 7.

42. De Souza Pereira, R. Regression of gastroesophageal reflux disease symptoms using dietary supplementation with melatonin, vitamins and aminoacids: Comparison with omeprazole. *J. Pineal. Res.* **2006**, *41*, 195–200.

43. Appleton, R.E.; Jones, A.P.; Gamble, C.; Williamson, P.R.; Wiggs, L.; Montgomery, P.; Sutcliffe, A.; Barker, C.; Gringras, P. The use of MElatonin in children with neurodevelopmental disorders and impaired sleep: A randomised, double-blind, placebo-controlled, parallel study (MENDS). *Health Technol. Assess.* **2012**, *16*, i-239.

44. Gringras, P.; Gamble, C.; Jones, A.P.; Wiggs, L.; Williamson, P.R.; Sutcliffe, A.; Montgomery, P.; Whitehouse, W.P.; Choonara, I.; Allport, T.; *et al.* Melatonin for sleep problems in children with neurodevelopmental disorders: Randomised double masked placebo controlled trial. *BMJ* **2012**, *345*, e6664.

45. Bendz, L.M.; Scates, A.C. Melatonin treatment for insomnia in pediatric patients with attention-deficit/hyperactivity disorder. *Ann. Pharmacother.* **2010**, *44*, 185–191.

46. Dickman, R.; Green, C.; Fass, S.S.; Quan, S.F.; Dekel, R.; Risner-Adler, S.; Fass, R. Relationships between sleep quality and pH monitoring findings in persons with gastroesophageal reflux disease. *J. Clin. Sleep Med.* **2007**, *3*, 505–513.

47. Ali, T. Sleep, immunity and inflammation in gastrointestinal disorders. *World J. Gastroenterol.* **2013**, *19*, 9231.

48. Dundee, J. P6 Acupressure and Postoperative Vomiting. *Br. J. Anaesth.* **1992**, *68*, 225–226.

49. Ezzo, J.M.; Richardson, M.A.; Vickers, A.; Allen, C.; Dibble, S.L.; Issell, B.F.; Lao, L.; Pearl, M.; Ramirez, G.; Roscoe, J.; *et al.* Acupuncture-point stimulation for chemotherapy-induced nausea or vomiting. *Cochrane Database Syst. Rev. Online* **2006**, doi:10.1002/14651858.CD002285.pub2.

50. McMillan, C.; Dundee, J. Enhancement of the antiemetic action of ondansetron by transcutaneous electrical stimulation of the P6 antiemetic point, in patients having highly emetic cytotoxic chemotherapy. *Br. J. Cancer* **1991**, *64*, 971–972.

51. Yeh, C.H.; Chien, L.-C.; Chiang, Y.C.; Lin, S.W.; Huang, C.K.; Ren, D. Reduction in nausea and vomiting in children undergoing cancer chemotherapy by either appropriate or sham auricular acupuncture points with standard care. *J. Altern. Complement. Med.* **2012**, *18*, 334–340.

52. Gottschling, S.; Reindl, T.; Meyer, S.; Berrang, J.; Henze, G.; Graeber, S.; Ong, M.F.; Graf, N. Acupuncture to alleviate chemotherapy-induced nausea and vomiting in pediatric oncology—A randomized multicenter crossover pilot trial. *Klin. Pädiatr.* **2008**, *220*, 365–370.

53. Reindl, T.K.; Geilen, W.; Hartmann, R.; Wiebelitz, K.R.; Kan, G.; Wilhelm, I.; Lugauer, S.; Behrens, C.; Weiberlenn, T.; Hasan, C.; *et al.* Acupuncture against chemotherapy-induced nausea and vomiting in pediatric oncology. Interim results of a multicenter crossover study. *Support Care Cancer* **2006**, *14*, 172–176.

54. Rusy, L.M.; Hoffman, G.M.; Weisman, S.J. Electroacupuncture prophylaxis of postoperative nausea and vomiting following pediatric tonsillectomy with or without adenoidectomy. *Anesthesiology* **2002**, *96*, 300–305.

55. Bai, L.; Yan, H.; Li, L.; Qin, W.; Chen, P.; Liu, P.; Gong, Q.; Liu, Y.; Tian, J. Neural specificity of acupuncture stimulation at pericardium 6: Evidence from an FMRI study. *J. Magn. Reson. Imaging* **2010**, *31*, 71–77.

56. Takahashi, T. Acupuncture for functional gastrointestinal disorders. *J. Gastroenterol.* **2006**, *41*, 408–417.

57. Jindal, V.; Ge, A.; Mansky, P.J. Safety and efficacy of acupuncture in children. *J. Pediatr. Hematol. Oncol.* **2008**, *30*, 431–442.

58. Jones, M.P.; Sharp, L.K.; Crowell, M.D. Psychosocial correlates of symptoms in functional dyspepsia. *Clin. Gastroenterol. Hepatol.* **2005**, *3*, 521–528.

59. Talley, N.J.; Boyce, P.; Jones, M. Dyspepsia and health care seeking in a community: How important are psychological factors? *Dig. Dis. Sci.* **1998**, *43*, 1016–1022.

60. Webb, A.N.; Kukuruzovic, R.H.; Catto-Smith, A.G.; Sawyer, S.M. Hypnotherapy for treatment of irritable bowel syndrome. *Cochrane Database Syst. Rev. Online* **2007**, doi:10.1002/14651858.CD005110.pub2.

61. Calvert, E.L.; Houghton, L.A.; Cooper, P.; Morris, J.; Whorwell, P.J. Long-term improvement in functional dyspepsia using hypnotherapy. *Gastroenterology* **2002**, *123*, 1778–1785.

62. Chiarioni, G.; Heymen, S.; Whitehead, W.E. Biofeedback therapy for dyssynergic defecation. *World J. Gastroenterol.* **2006**, *12*, 7069–7074.

63. Van Tilburg, M.A.L.; Chitkara, D.K.; Palsson, O.S.; Turner, M.; Blois-Martin, N.; Ulshen, M.; Whitehead, W.E. Audio-recorded guided imagery treatment reduces functional abdominal pain in children: A pilot study. *Pediatrics* **2009**, *124*, e890–e897.

64. Weydert, J.A.; Shapiro, D.E.; Acra, S.A.; Monheim, C.J.; Chambers, A.S.; Ball, T.M. Evaluation of guided imagery as treatment for recurrent abdominal pain in children: A randomized controlled trial. *BMC Pediatr.* **2006**, *6*, 29.

65. Vlieger, A.M.; Menko-Frankenhuis, C.; Wolfkamp, S.C.S.; Tromp, E.; Benninga, M.A. Hypnotherapy for children with functional abdominal pain or irritable bowel syndrome: A randomized controlled trial. *Gastroenterology* **2007**, *133*, 1430–1436.

66. Rutten, J.M.T.M.; Reitsma, J.B.; Vlieger, A.M.; Benninga, M.A. Gut-directed hypnotherapy for functional abdominal pain or irritable bowel syndrome in children: A systematic review. *Arch. Dis. Child.* **2013**, *98*, 252–257.

67. El-Serag, H. Role of obesity in GORD-related disorders. *Gut* **2008**, *57*, 281–284.

68. Jacobson, B.C.; Somers, S.C.; Fuchs, C.S.; Kelly, C.P.; Camargo, C.A., Jr. Body-mass index and symptoms of gastroesophageal reflux in women. *N. Engl. J. Med.* **2006**, *354*, 2340–2348.

69. Ness-Jensen, E.; Lindam, A.; Lagergren, J.; Hveem, K. Weight loss and reduction in gastroesophageal reflux. A prospective population-based cohort study: The HUNT study. *Am. J. Gastroenterol.* **2013**, *108*, 376–382.

Clinical Hypnosis with Children and Adolescents—What? Why? How?: Origins, Applications, and Efficacy

Daniel P. Kohen and Pamela Kaiser

Abstract: This review article addresses the process, intention, and therapeutic value of clinical hypnosis with children and adolescents. A brief historical perspective is followed by a digest of the published laboratory and clinical research that has accelerated substantially over the past two decades. This review lends appropriate credence to the benefits and integration to clinical practice of this powerful tool for teaching young people self-regulation skills. The breadth of application is described, and several clinical vignettes are provided as examples of what is possible. In addition to the provision of the most relevant citations in the pediatric, psychological, and neuroscience literature, this synopsis concludes with information regarding availability of skill development training in pediatric clinical hypnosis.

Reprinted from *Children*. Cite as: Kohen, D.P.; Kaiser, P. Clinical Hypnosis with Children and Adolescents—What?Why? How?: Origins, Applications, and Efficacy. *Children* **2014**, *1*, 74-98.

1. Introduction

The review that follows is designed to be a panoramic snapshot of the current state of the art, science, and clinical practice of child hypnosis and hypnotherapy. While substantial reference resource material is provided and clinical examples described, this is nonetheless a synopsis, and readers are advised and strongly encouraged to consult the resources and to avail themselves of "hands-on" skill-development workshop training to develop skills necessary to begin helping children with clinical hypnosis.

The field of pediatric hypnosis has blossomed in many ways and directions over time:

- From a backdrop focus on societal and cultural beliefs and norms to a context of fostering respect for the child's creativity, imagination, unique perceptions, and choices.
- From the view of hypnosis as a ritual completed by an authority figure *on* the individual to an interactive, dynamic "dance-like" experience *between* two individuals, with the clinician sometimes "leading" and other times "pacing" while the child leads.
- From the use, writings, and research by a select group of clinicians, *i.e.*, physicians and psychologists, to the broadened utilization by and contributions from various types of health care providers with advanced degrees.
- From apprenticeship learning at the bedside of highly specified hypnotic techniques to the richness of multi-modal and multi-sensory training within a group setting, based on research about adult learning and skill acquisition, emphasizing the multiple paths toward similar clinical goals.
- From definitions based on the fixed views and narrow theoretical concepts of a few to the fertile exchange by many within a global community.

- From precise suggested commands applied rigidly to *all* patients to open-ended, permissive, and *individualized* suggestions utilizing the specific needs, resources, and interests of each child or teen.
- From making conclusions and generalizations about the hypnotic experience based solely on behavioral observation to incorporating double-blind research studies evaluated in Cochrane reviews and state-of-the-art neuroimaging to correlate with the varying types of hypnotic behavior.

2. Brief History of Hypnosis & Hypnosis with Children

In ancient times hypnotic-like techniques were utilized in healing and other ceremonies [1]. (Biblical references in both the Old and New Testaments describe accounts of ill children responding to healing methods based on faith and suggestion (I Kings XVII: 17–24; Mark IX: 17–27). Primitive cultures have employed trance phenomena with children in initiation rites and other ceremonies [1].

The modern history of hypnosis—in both children and adults—can be found in the rich, fascinating, and challenging history of many physicians of 18th century Europe and even more so in the 19th century. Many physicians contributed substantial clinical experience and theoretical concepts to our current understanding of clinical hypnosis and its usefulness in clinical health care. Amongst many, these included Franz Anton Mesmer (1734–1815), the British Surgeon John Elliotson (1791–1868) who also introduced the stethoscope to Great Britain, James Braid (1795–1860) who coined the word hypnosis, and Jean-Martin Charcot (1835–1893) whose descriptions of hypnosis in neurological terms gave it a new measure of scientific respectability. Of import, Liebault (1823–1904) and Bernheim (1840–1919) founded the School of Nancy devoted to the scientific investigation of hypnosis and described the first research on children's hypnotic susceptibility, describing over 750 subjects and the peak "susceptibility" thought in those days to occur between the ages of 7 and 14 years [2] (Kohen and Olness, 2011; pp. 7–12).

A more detailed description of the early history of hypnosis with children is beyond the scope of this article and can be found in Kohen and Olness' text Hypnosis and Hypnotherapy with Children (4th edition, 2011) [2].

Kohen and Olness (2011) note the apparent beginning of child hypnosis in the U.S. [2] with Baldwin's paper entitled "Suggestion in Infancy" in *Science* published in 1891 [3]. By 1900, interest in child hypnosis in Europe and the U.S. had decreased and it was not until the late 1950s and early 1960s that there was a resurgence of interest in research in Child Hypnosis. In the late 1950s psychiatrists Dr. Milton Erickson [4] and Dr. M. Erik Wright [5] described their clinical use of hypnosis/hypnotherapy with children.

In the 1960s Dr. Franz Baumann, a general pediatrician in San Francisco, was the first pediatrician to become President of a major Hypnosis Society (The American Society of Clinical Hypnosis). He published papers on the applications of hypnosis for adolescent drug abuse, enuresis, and encopresis [6,7]. In that decade several so-called Susceptibility Scales for Hypnotic Susceptibility in Children were developed (London and Cooper, 1969, [8]; Barber & Calverley, 1963, [9]). The "gold standard" for hypnotic susceptibility in children, the Stanford Children's

Hypnotic Susceptibility Scale (used primarily in research) was developed and published in 1979 by Arlene Morgan, Ph.D. & Josephine Hilgard, Ph.D. (see Kohen and Olness, 2011, appendix) [2].

Additional clinical reports emerged in the 1970s, most notably by G. Gail Gardner, Ph.D. [10], Karen Olness, M.D., the acknowledged pioneer and "mother of pediatric clinical hypnosis" [11], and Lonnie Zeltzer, M.D. and Sam LeBaron, M.D, Ph.D. who did early and important clinical and research work with pediatric oncology patients [12–14], The first formal workshop in child hypnosis was taught in 1976 at the International Congress of Hypnosis in Philadelphia [15].

The first textbook, Hypnosis and Hypnotherapy with Children, was written by G. Gail Gardner, Ph.D. and Karen Olness, M.D. and published in 1981 [16]. The second edition was published in 1988 [17], the third in 1996 by Karen Olness, M.D. and Daniel P. Kohen, M.D. [18], and the most recent, fourth edition in 2011 by Kohen and Olness [2]. The third edition was also translated into and published in German [19] and French [20].

Beyond milestones noted in Table 1 [21–32], many clinical applications of hypnosis in child health began to be reported in the 1980s and increasingly in the 1990s, notably clinical and research papers on the efficacy and applications for clinical hypnosis for children with asthma [33,34], children with cancer [14,22–25] and tic and Tourette Syndrome [35].

Following the aforementioned initial pediatric clinical hypnosis training workshop in 1976, occasional half-day to two day advanced workshops in pediatric hypnosis were offered to experienced child health clinicians sporadically during annual conferences of the American Society of Clinical Hypnosis (ASCH) and the Society for Clinical and Experimental Hypnosis (SCEH). Beginning in 1987, annual 3-day pediatric hypnosis workshops were offered under the auspices of the American organization, the Society for Developmental-Behavioral Pediatrics (SDBP), as part of its annual meeting. Given this workshop's wonderful success the following year concurrent Introductory *and* Intermediate Level training workshops were offered, and an Advanced Pediatric Clinical Hypnosis Workshop was added the next year. These three concurrent workshops were provided annually through 2009. Beginning in 2010, the Faculty from these preceding 24 years remained together and the National Pediatric Hypnosis Training Institute (NPHTI) was co-founded by Daniel Kohen, MD and Pamela Kaiser, PhD, CPNP, CNS. By Fall, 2014, NPHTI's 5th annual tri-level workshops will have tripled their faculty in order to meet the growing attendance by multi-disciplinary clinicians from around the globe.

Kindertagung—the Child Hypnosis Congress—is the largest child hypnosis congress in the world, due to the vision of organizer and teacher, Bernhard Trenkle, Dipl. Psych. and Director of the Milton Erickson Institute in Rottweil, Germany. It was established initially in 1990 in Rottweil, and attracted 300 participants. Two years later, it was offered by a larger faculty in Heidelberg, Germany, and over 450 attended. Over the next sixteen years, it was offered four additional times with continued exponential growth in attendance. In 2013 the 7th Kindertagung was held in Heidelberg , with 2000 attendees including 114 faculty from Germany, France, Italy, Switzerland, South Africa, Canada, and the U.S. [32].

Table 1. Key Milestones in 20th–21st Century Evolution of Pediatric Hypnosis.

Year	Milestone	Comment/Reference
1984	Largest clinical series (to date) of Pediatric patients treated with Hypnosis	[21] Kohen, D.P., Olness, K.N., Colwell, S., & Heimel
1986 & 1999	Seminal Videos produced documenting the value of hypnosis in children with Cancer: "No Fears, No Tears" and the sequel "No Fears, No Tears- 13 years later"	[22,23] Leora Kuttner, Ph.D. Vancouver, BC Canada [24,25]
1987 (to 2009)	First Annual Workshops in Pediatric Clinical Hypnosis for Child Health Clinicians–under auspices of Society for Developmental and Behavioral Pediatrics	[2] Inaugural in Disneyland 1987 under auspices of SDBP Annually 1987–2009.
1989	First Pediatric Psychoneuroimmunology study	[26]
1997	"Imaginative Medicine – Hypnosis in Pediatric Practice "Video documenting value of hypnosis in primary care	[27] Laurence I. Sugarman, M.D. Rochester Institute of Technology, Rochester NY
2005, 2009	Harry the Hypno-potamus: Metaphorical Tales for Pediatric Problems (Vol I 2005, Vol II in 2009)	[28,29] Linda Thomson, CPNP
1996, 2011	Hypnosis and Hypnotherapy with Children published 3rd edition 1996, 4th edition 2011	[2,18] 3rd ed Olness KN and Kohen, DP 1996 4th ed Kohen, DP and Olness, KN 2011
2007—2nd ed 2013	Therapeutic Hypnosis with Children and Adolescents published 1st edition 2007 and 2nd edition 2014	[30] Editors: WC Wester and LI Sugarman 2007 2nd ed: Sugarman & Wester 2014
2010 (annual)	**Formation of NPHTI—National Pediatric Hypnosis Training Institute** -Inaugural Annual Skill Development Workshops in Pediatric Clinical Hypnosis (Introductory, Intermediate and Advanced) **www.nphti.com**	[31] Co-Founders and Co-Directors Pamela Kaiser, PhD, CPNP, CNS Daniel P. Kohen, MD, FAAP, ABMH 2010–2014 and ongoing **www.nphti.com**
2010	"Non-pharmacological treatment of tics in Tourette Syndrome with videotape training in self-hypnosis." *JDBP*	[2] (p 310) Lazarus and Klein article including link to video illustration of hypnosis with a child with Tourette Syndrome.
1990, 1992, 1997, 2002, 2005, 2009, 2013	Kindertagung = Largest Child Hypnosis Congress *in the world*—begun 1990, most recent Heidelberg Germany, 2013	[32] Bernhard Trenkle, Dipl Psych

3. Definition

Over the past three decades professionals have proposed a variety of theoretical definitions based upon controlled clinical laboratory research [36].

The American Society of Clinical Hypnosis provides the following definition on its website (www.asch.net):

> *"**Definition of Hypnosis:** Hypnosis is a state of inner absorption, concentration and focused attention. It is like using a magnifying glass to focus the rays of the sun and make them more powerful. Similarly, when our minds are concentrated and focused, we are able to use our minds more powerfully. Because hypnosis allows people to use more of their potential, learning self-hypnosis is the ultimate act of self-control.... Recent research supports the view that hypnotic communication and suggestions effectively changes aspects of the persons physiological and neurological functions."*

The American Psychological Association Division 30 states in their 2014 revised official definition [37].

> ***Hypnosis** is a state of consciousness involving focused attention and reduced peripheral awareness characterized by an enhanced capacity for response to suggestion; **hypnotizability** is an individual's ability to experience suggested alterations in physiology, sensations, emotions, thoughts, or behavior during hypnosis; and **hypnotherapy**: The use of hypnosis in the treatment of a medical or psychological disorder or concern.*

OR, as pediatrician Laurence Sugarman added his perspective [38] (Sugarman, NPHTI presentation, September 2013).

> *"When we are IN hypnosis, we intensify our attention, decrease our peripheral awareness and become more receptive to new ideas and associations whenever we reinforce, rewire, reframe or otherwise alter the neurophysiological networks we call "experience". Trance is what happens when we engage in changing our minds."* He goes on to say that *"Hypnosis is about creating therapeutic interpersonal space for trance-formation that leads to transformation."* [38] and, provides a definition that says that *"Hypnosis is A skill set involving interpersonal communication designed to facilitate therapeutic change in maladaptive psycho- physiological reflexes."* [38] *(Otherwise, of course, WHY do it?!)*

More recently theories and definitions have been proposed based upon neurophysiological research aimed precisely at identifying and describing the neurophysiologic correlates of hypnotic behavior, reported and observed hypnotic features and effects, now verified with the availability and use of functional MRI (fMRI), PET scans, and related physiologic measures [39,40] *etc.*

Using brain imaging, cognitive neuroscientists have identified the power that suggestions have over attention functions and associated brain networks and their impact on physical and mental experience.

(Raz, 2011, [40]). Still, Amir Raz, a leader in the field of neurohypnosis, cautions about the common over-interpretation of fMRI findings. He notes that researchers are now using newer techniques combined with fMRIs in the goal of identifying brain regions associated with different cognitive functions [40] We await further exciting discoveries from these and other researchers.

The most recent issue of Mind-Body-Regulation [41] (MBR, 5 May 2014) brought together the world's most distinguished scholars to create a decisive definition of hypnosis that has eluded scholars over the past century. While they provided stimulating food for thought, they did not reach a mutually agreed upon conclusion or provide a unifying definition [41].

Although there is no universally agreed-upon or scientifically validated definition of hypnosis, we prefer a descriptive definition that elucidates what we believe to be the fundamental ingredients of the hypnotic experience and phenomenon from a clinical perspective/in a clinical setting:

> *A spontaneously occurring or induced alternative state of awareness (with or without relaxation, which may or may not be evident) in which an individual develops a focused concentration on some idea or image with the expressed purpose of maximizing potential, creating a CHANGE, and/or reducing or resolving some problem [2] (Kohen and Olness, 2011).*

4. What is It?

Building on the preceding purposes delineated in the definition by Kohen and Olness, we would like to expand our conceptualization of clinical pediatric hypnosis as a tool to facilitate the evolution and refinement of **self-regulation skills and capacities**. More specifically, hypnosis is a tool to strengthen children's existing or under-developed skills in self-regulation, *i.e.*, capacities to *shift attention*, maintain *focused attention*, inhibit and control reflexive actions, delay gratification, use problem solving strategies, and self-monitor and modulate thinking, emotion, behavior, and psycho-physiological reactivity [42]. Children typically develop this capacity during infancy and childhood [43]. With appropriate clinical pediatric hypnosis training, child health clinicians can help children and youth to identify, discover, develop, and cultivate these capacities and other internal resources for their own benefit in managing and shaping their responses to a broad range of health and life problems, dilemmas, and challenges [42]. In this regard clinical hypnosis helps children and their parents develop and refine the concept of "skills not pills" [44] as strategies to apply to their particular problems or concerns.

We wish to emphasize that we believe that the critical ingredients of the therapeutic hypnotic experience in children (as well as in adults) are focused attention to and absorption in imagination which includes a focus on multi-sensory imagery and a particular *cultivation of that imagination* on steps and strategies toward goals for resolution of problems and change of ineffective patterns. Examples of possible specific goals include diminution or disappearance of undesirable symptoms, accurate discrimination of distorted thinking about situations and stressors, re-framing of perception of problems as solvable and conditions as manageable, building positive expectations, control of exaggerated reactivity, and creation and enhancement of the belief in the ability of the mind and body to work together to evoke and create desirable changes in outcome.

While this is not the forum for an expanded discussion of the similarities and differences between hypnosis and other self-regulatory activities, we are aware of other modalities that incorporate experiential learning and mechanisms for change. We are clear in telling our clients and patients that "some people call this work hypnosis, some call it imagery, some call it visualization, others refer to it as mindfulness, and some call it biofeedback." We indicate our belief that these approaches bear some similarity to one another and may reflect some overlap of the same phenomenology. These activities share the goals of helping people to cultivate internal resources, to explore new possibilities, to accomplish physiologic, perceptual, sensory, and behavioral changes, and to facilitate mind-body communication and modulation [45–47].

5. Why Use Hypnosis? Why Do It?

In a video prepared by one of us (DK) for teaching clinicians how children understand and apply self-hypnosis [48] an eleven-year-old boy with Asthma who improved substantially with the application of his self-hypnosis skills is asked "**How** does **your** hypnosis help you with your asthma?" He begins by saying "How does it help the medicine work better and faster? Yeah, it does, I don't know how. How does it help me feel better… breathe easier? Well, ummmmm, uhhh, it's kind of hard to explain….." and then turns his face to the camera and says, "Well, it works….. okay, all you people out there, it works!" This clinical evidence is followed below by a review of the published evidence.

6. Wide Spectrum of Applications

As described in the historical review, the beginning of a surge of clinical reports and clinical research in pediatric hypnosis began in the 1970s and continues today. This substantive increase may be causally related—and certainly temporally related—to the concurrent evolution of increased workshop training in pediatric clinical hypnosis during these decades as discussed above.

In 1984 Kohen and colleagues published what remains today the largest clinical series of children (505 children) and youth treated with hypnosis for a variety of clinical problems, including enuresis, pain, asthma, habit disorders, obesity, encopresis, and anxiety [21]. In 1987 Olness, Uden and McDonald published their seminal research documenting the superiority of hypnosis training to medication in the treatment of juvenile migraine [49].

In appropriate search of physiologic correlates of the hypnotic experience in children, studies have been conducted describing changes found in peripheral skin temperature during hypnosis [50], in transcutaneous oxygen flux [51], cardiovascular changes in association with hypnosis [52,53], pulmonary function changes in children with asthma learning hypnosis [34,54].

The value of hypnosis in modulating the negative effects of chemotherapy for children with cancer (such as nausea and vomiting) has been demonstrated in the research and clinical work of Zeltzer and LeBaron [12–14], Olness [55], Jacknow and colleagues [56], and dramatically in Kuttner's award-winning educational videos "No Fears, No Tears" and "No Fears, No Tears—13 years Later" [22,23] 1986, and Making Every Moment Count [25]. Kohen and Zajac recently described the efficacy of hypnosis for headaches in children and teens [57]. Subsequently Kohen reported an important follow-up survey demonstrating the long-term benefits of hypnosis for those who had originally benefited from learning hypnosis for relief of headaches and reported not only long-term sustained relief, but also the application of those skills to other areas of their lives [58]. Recently, Sugarman and colleagues have published an award-winning article describing new theories and promising research regarding the value of hypnosis (and biofeedback) with young people with autism [59].

In recent years the increase in use of clinical hypnosis with children has resulted in a plethora of publications for a wide variety of clinical problems. For example, in preparation of the fourth edition of Hypnosis and Hypnotherapy with Children (2011) [2] the authors reviewed over 500 newly published articles from the English, French, and German literature, published since the third edition in 1996 [18].

For a detailed and wide-ranging description of the myriad of clinical conditions for which hypnosis is applicable and effective in children and youth, readers are encouraged to consult the two standard texts in this field, Kohen and Olness' 2011 fourth edition Hypnosis the Hypnotherapy with Children [2] and Sugarman and Wester's edited text, Therapeutic Hypnosis with Children and Adolescents, second edition (2014) [30].

Additionally, we refer to the following Table 2 that highlights a broad range of applications.

Table 2. Applications of Hypnotherapy for Children and Adolescents *.

Category	Examples	Key References
1. Habit Problems	Thumb-sucking, nail-biting, Hair-pulling, Nocturnal Enuresis, Habit Cough	GGailGardner 1978 [10] D Kohen 1996 [60] L Thomson (2002) [61] Gottsegen (2003) [62] Anbar and Hall (2004) [63] Shenefelt (2004) [64] Anbar (2007) [65] Olness (1975) [11]
2. Mental Health Conditions	Separation Anxiety • Social Anxiety • Performance Anxiety (speeches, recital, sports) • post traumatic stress disorder (PTSD) • obsessive compulsive disorder (OCD) • Phobias Grief & Bereavement Major Depression • Dysthymia • Adjustment Disorder with Depression and Anxiety Anger • Adjustment Disorder • Coping with family change	Kaiser (2011) [42] Kaiser (2014) [94] Spies (1979) [95] Kuttner, Friedrichsdorf (2014) [96] Golden (2012) [97] Kerns et al (2013) [98] Yapko (2001) [99] Yapko (2006) [100] Yapko (2011) [70] Kohen, Murray (2006) [101] Kohen (2014) [102] Cyr, Culbert, Kaiser 2003 [66] Tschann, Kaiser, Boyce, Chesney, Alkon-Leonard (1996) [67] Culbert & R-Cyr, Ped Mind-Body Interface (2005) [68] Olness (2009) [69] Yapko (2011) [70]

Table 2. *Cont.*

Category	Examples	Key References
3. Psycho-Physiological Disorders	Asthma • Migraine HA •IBS Inflammatory Bowel Disease • Warts • Tourette Syndrome	Kohen & Zajac 2007 [57] Kohen (2010, 2011) [58,71] Olness, MacDonald Uden (1987) [44] LaBaw (1975) [72] Anbar (2003) [73] Hackman (2000) [74] Kohen (1995) [33] Kohen, Wynne (1997) [34] Culbert, Kajander, Kohen Reaney (1996) [75] Gottsegen (2011) [76] Kuttner et al (2006) [77] Vlieger, Menko-Frankenhuis (2007) [78] Pendergrast (2003) [79] Lazarus, Klein (2010) [2] (p. 310) Kohen, Botts (1987) [35]
4. Pain	Acute (injury, illness, medical procedures) • Chronic pain • Recurrent Pain	Kohen (1995) [80] Kuttner (2006) [81] Olness (1981) [50] Berberich, Landman (2009) [82] Myers, Bergman, Zeltzer (2004) [83] Zeltzer, Dolgin, LeBaron, S., LeBaon, C. (1991) [84] Vlieger, Menko-Frankenhuis (2007) [78] Gottsegen (2011) [76] Anbar (2001) [85] Antich (1967) [86] Bernstein (1965) [87] Butler et al (2005) [88] French, GM et al (1994) [89] Kohen, (1996) [90] Kuttner (1988) [24] Kuttner (2010) [91] LeBaron, Hilgard (1984) [14] Tsao, *et al.*, (2007) [92] Uman et al (2008) [93] Gulewitsch, Muller, Hutzinger, Schlarb (2013) [109]
5. Sleep Disorders	Sleep onset insomnia (Anx), Circadian Rhythm Disorder, Parasomnias	Culbert, Kajander (2007) [103] Kuttner (2009) [104] Kaiser (2011) [42] Kohen et al (1996) [105] Stanton (1989) [106] Schlarb, Liddle, Hautzinger (2011) [110]

Table 2. *Cont.*

Category	Examples	Key References
6. Chronic Illness	Adjustment & coping Palliative Care, Grief, Bereavement	Anbar (2000) [54] Anbar (2001) [85] Zeltzer, Schlank (2005) [107] Kuttner, Friedrichsdorf (2014), [96] Kuttner (2006), [81] Kuttner (2003), [25] Kohen, Olness (2011, Chapter 15) [2] Gardner (1976) [108] *

* While several illustrative references are cited, additional relevant examples and references can be found in the two major textbooks, noted in references [2,30].

The value of brain imaging in amplifying how hypnotic suggestions impact mental and physical experience is described by Lifshitz, Cusumano, and Raz (2013) [111]. It is also noteworthy that Cochrane and other systematic reviews support the efficacy of pediatric hypnosis for various clinical applications, including Curtis *et al.*, (2012) [112], Gold *et al.*, (2007) [113], Landier & Tse (2010) [114], McClaffery (2011) [115], Rickardson *et al.*, (2006) [116], Schnur *et al.*, (2008) [117], and Uman *et al.*, (2013) [118].

7. Case Presentations

The remainder of this paper offers several case vignettes to illustrate common applications of hypnosis and hypnotherapy in every-day child and adolescent health care. These case examples also demonstrate the nature and value of these empowering hypnosis strategies for children who previously struggled substantially before developing various self-regulation skills:

7.1. Case of Anxiety

7.1.1. CASE #1: Performance Anxiety: From Baseball Bawling to Behavioral and Emotional Self-Regulation

J. is a 9-year-old fourth grader who presented with a long history of anxiety about not measuring up to his own very high standards. This was associated with poor emotional and behavioral self-regulation when frustrated and disappointed with his mistakes, which was particularly detrimental when playing his beloved sport, baseball. Despite his Dad's coaching tricks to let go of these feelings, he typically needed to be assisted off the pitcher's mound due to uncontrollable tears, kicking the dirt, and hitting himself with his glove. He was unable to "regroup" from this marked emotional and behavioral disintegration and the sobbing continued, resulting in reduced playing time, embarrassment, and later regret and further anxiety.

As with all initial encounters with new patients, developing rapport with the child and parents is critical to the process and outcome of the treatment. Similarly, the clinician learns the child's personal and family history, and assesses motivation, expectations, strengths and other internal resources, such as capacity to accurately discriminate or interpret a situation and to self-regulate their emotions, thoughts, and behavior in other areas of their life. Time is spent to appraise the child's understanding of the "problem" as well as *how* they accomplished past mastery experiences.

While there may be some exceptions, the more formalized introduction of hypnosis *per se* and discussion and demystification of hypnosis may not take place until subsequent visit(s). Given this child's strong interest in sports, the clinician linked the explanation about hypnosis to references about top athletes' learned skills in focused attention, mental rehearsal, and being "in the zone". She emphasized that "learning to do 'self-hypnosis' like those athletes do will certainly help his game".

Children in this age range are particularly receptive and responsive to hypnosis. The clinician capitalizes on this developmental phase, by utilizing the child's expanded attention span, intellectual curiosity, motivation to master new skills, capacity to understand and create metaphors, and the ability to access memories of the past and to richly imagine the future.

This child saw his "hypnosis coach" weekly for several sessions, during which hypnosis was incorporated into other interventions, including Cognitive Behavior Therapy (CBT) to address his faulty beliefs and perfectionism, computerized biofeedback to enhance his psycho-physiological reactivity, and parent counseling to shift from their sense of helplessness to learning how to support their son's own growing capacities to dampen strong emotions. He also kept a calendar to record his improving self-regulation skills, using a scale from 0 to 10 to indicate level of control over behavioral outbursts.

When designing a hypnotic or hypnosis trance experience, the clinician "utilizes" the child's interests, capacities, and goals. J's notable strengths included his passion and knowledge of baseball, his overall congenial personality and sportsmanship, and his motivation to gain self-control. Given his pronounced passion for baseball, the child and therapist made an agreement: He would teach her baseball terms and she would teach him "tricks" to improve his self-control and focus during baseball games. Accordingly, sports terminology, the self-calming rituals of his favorite star ball players, and his capacity to focus his attention were incorporated into therapeutic suggestions. In this regard, J. was asked to "teach" the clinician about sports slang and to tell some stories about key players. This language and information became "hooks" woven into suggestions during the hypnosis work.

For example, the phrase "on to the next one!" was introduced to J. as self-talk, an immediate inner response, to dissociate from any personal errors during the game and to sustain positive expectations. He also learned to "turn off the faucets" just before each practice and game, in order to control his past tearful responses and to regulate his intense emotional reactivity to mistakes. While he imagined playing a close game, he was taught to pair or link a calming breath with the touch of the ball when pitching, bat when hitting, and base when running.

He was also told a metaphoric story about a boy who decided it was time to no longer feel like a *loser* by being tricked by *curve balls* inside his head that were *stealing* his attention, focus and control. First, he found a *specialty coach* to work with on his *mental game* during his *spring training* and he found immediate *relief* with the *assist* of calming breaths. Second, he taught himself to *throw* away any *errors* that were *running around* in his head, in order to quickly *catch* on to practicing new *plays*. Third, he worked hard on *drills* to *line up* his new strategies in his mind. Before the end of his inner strength training, he *struck out* the old disappointment and frustration that had *fouled* up his *game*. He became a *champion* as a *triple threat* with his MVP—Most Valuable Playing—with full attention, focus, and self-control. *Watch him keeping his eyes on the ball, instead of bawling!*

This story was recorded and given to him, with instructions to listen to it daily as part of his ongoing practice doing self-hypnosis exercises to foster calmness and an enhanced capacity to modulate his emotions when coping with normal, every day "hassles". In subsequent sessions, the clinician reviewed his progress calendar and added other hypnosis experiences for him to listen to daily.

Within a number of weeks, this child showed significantly enhanced self-regulation of his emotions and behavior, both on and off the field. He became an athlete who shared his self-control strategies with his teammates.

7.1.2. CASE #2: Anger Management and Primary Nocturnal Enuresis

Almost 10-year-old "Z" was brought by his parents for "issues" of angry behavior and not wanting to do what he is told or asked, occurring exclusively at home. He has had no problems in school or in after-school programs, but acknowledged "issues" with stomping his feet, slamming doors, and defiantly refusing to do things he is "supposed" to do at home, either on his own or when asked.

The day before his first visit he had a public tantrum at a local store when his mother said he could not get the toy he wanted. As a "consequence" of his tantrum, he was "grounded" from using his electronic games for a week. His mother reported that she was surprised that he had spontaneously come to her to apologize that same evening before bed. He was surprised and proud when the clinician spontaneously gave him a "high 5!" for that spontaneous apology.

During the initial visit the clinician inquired what "issues" Z wanted to work on. He said he did not like the way he gets angry and was surprised when the clinician told him that "feeling angry is okay, everyone I ever met got angry or gets angry sometimes, and then they get un-angry. It is only okay or not okay *how* we get angry and *how* we act, not *if* we get angry. We are not allowed to hurt people or things when we get *angry*. The clinician noted Z's spontaneous focused attention (spontaneous hypnotic trance) and complimented *all those other times that you might have gotten angry and did not.*

During the first visit the clinician identified Z's strengths, including cooperation at school (*i.e.*, no behavior problems or acting out there), great soccer skills, and being a "quick learner".

Almost as an after-thought Z. mentioned that he had an "issue" with his bladder and he and his parents noted that he *never* wakes up in a dry bed. When asked about the *reason* for this, they said "because he sleeps too soundly, he's a heavy, deep sleeper". When he told the clinician that there was no problem with daytime wetting *ever*, the clinician purposely and dramatically showed pleasant surprise: "*really*? Well, that's going to make this *much easier to solve* than I thought, we'll work on this as soon as you know how to manage the *angry* feelings." This "waking hypnotic suggestion" was planted as a seed for building upon at a future visit.

At the second visit, Z. was taught a hypnotic anger (or other feeling) management strategy called the "jettison technique". Offering a "personal" example, the clinician gave a blank piece of paper to Z. and one for himself. Without formally mentioning hypnosis, the clinician said "Just listen and watch first. Then you'll have a chance to *do* this too… Sometimes when I feel angry I just close my eyes or I look inside my mind with my eyes *open*—either way is fine—and I picture what *color and shape* angry is…. Let's see, hmmmm, right now it's a *red square*! Then, I imagine or pretend there is a faucet or drain pipe in the side of that square. I turn it on and the angry feeling runs out of my thinking (touching each next part while describing it) down the side of my neck, down my shoulder on my (either) arm and down and around the bend at the elbow and all the way down into the palm of my hand (holding palm upward) until all of the angry feeling has filled up my hand. Then I roll it up into a tight fist, take a deep breath and hold it, then as I blow out *I throw it away*!! (forcibly crumpling up the piece of paper as tight as possible and throwing it onto the floor!). At the end, I look *back* into my thinking to see the *color and shape of comfortable or relief or relaxed*…wow, now it's a yellow circle, smiley face!! Okay, your turn!" He reproduced it, reporting different colors and shapes than the clinician's. It was suggested that he have a pile of scrap paper in his room to use "as needed".

At the next visit he and his parents reported considerably fewer tantrums and much more cooperation. He asked about getting *dry* at night. He was told quite directly that his brain and bladder *know each other very well,* that they work together great, and are in a good *pattern* of talking to each other, so much so that he does not wet his pants *even* if he has to "go really, really badly…" He agreed, and said that what was just described was exactly what he *does* every day all day except that he does not say it *out loud.*

Z. demonstrated another spontaneous hypnotic state while focusing carefully on a participatory drawing of genitourinary anatomy and physiology, capitalizing on his curiosity about how the body works, and his quick learning.

In the drawing, urine was depicted being sent from the kidneys (aka "pee factory") to the bladder, shown as a "sack with a muscle around it" with a "gate" made of muscle that is closed most of the time, opening only upon signal from the "main computer", *i.e.*, the brain, when it is full. The drawing showed the brain and bladder connection, with bi-directional arrows communicating between the full bladder and the brain, keeping the gate "closed" until the right time and place.

Z. was taught that nighttime accidents are just that, *i.e.* that *his brain and bladder accidentally got into an accidental habit or pattern of not talking with each other at night.* Therefore, he has to remind them before he goes to sleep *because* he is going to be asleep. Since the bladder and brain have perfect communication all day long, they "are already friends and know how to talk to each other, so *all* you have to do is *remind them before you go to sleep.*"

Z. committed to giving instructions at bedtime to his brain and bladder "taking no longer than 5 min to do so". "For example, you could say "Bladder, tonight let the brain know when you're full. Brain, you have a choice: WHEN the bladder says it's full, tell me to wake up, walk to the bathroom, open the gate, pee in the toilet, close the gate, flush , and go back to my *nice, warm, comfortable dry bed*, or, instead *tell the bladder gate to stay closed and locked all night until morning*, and *then* wake up happy and proud in a nice warm dry bed" With either choice, the bed is dry in the morning.

Z listened carefully. His parents and he agreed to discontinue using "diapers" (pull-ups) that he had worn—and soaked—nightly. Although they missed the scheduled appointment 2 weeks later, they returned in 4 weeks to report 29 out of 32 nights being totally *dry*, or 91% dryness. His parents were astounded, and he was very proud.

7.1.3. Case #3: Fear of Shots and Embarrassing Warts

K. was a 10-year-old fifth grader who asked her parents to see the "special doctor" who helped her good friend get over daily tummy aches while at school when she was away from her Mom. K. wanted to get over her long-time fear of shots. She was also highly motivated to get rid of several large warts on her knees. She was tired of always wearing pants to cover them for fear of being teased.

The evaluation showed that her fear of injections met criteria for a Specific Phobia, given her excessive and developmentally inappropriate level of fear reactivity regarding the procedure. Her mother described K's intense distress and panic whenever faced with this procedure in the past. She begged loudly for a delay, tried to hide in the corner of the exam room, cried and screamed in protest when the nurse approached her. Her screeches "No! No! No!" lasted until some minutes after the administration.

Given her panic symptoms of high psychophysiological and emotional reactivity, K. was taught diaphragmatic breathing (aka "belly breathing") to activate the parasympathetic nervous system (aka the "calming control center, CCC"). She was urged to practice this new skill several times a day.

Because Exposure Therapy with Systematic Desensitization is the treatment of choice for phobias, K. was gradually exposed to the equipment (e.g., cleaning swab, syringe) and procedure for injections, until those items and "pretend" shot-giving no longer evoked activation of panic symptoms. In addition to this "*in vivo*" exposure, she was taught self-hypnosis to be used as repeated "imaginal exposure" that focused on her capacity for self-regulation of her body's "false alarm" that had prompted such strong reactions with her emotions, thoughts, and behavior.

Given her gift for creative writing and love of biographies about strong-willed girls who became famous women, she was encouraged to "go to a special *safe* place where she was completely in charge and in control of herself". She was invited to "just enjoy being *there* where she could also *now* turn on a special TV in her mind". Suggestions were offered "to use your imagination to watch a Mastery Movie on the K Channel. Instead of watching the *old* disaster film of being out of control while getting a shot, this is a '*future* film', you are the scriptwriter, the producer, the director, *and* the star of the show".

She was encouraged to use her five senses to intensify the experience "*as if* you are really there: calmly and confidently walking into the waiting room, becoming even more relaxed and completely in control as you enter the exam room. Now notice how easily you deepen your sense of calmness by using your belly breathing and self-hypnosis when the nurse comes in to *give* the medicine *that keeps you healthy*. Pay attention to how you go so quickly to your Special Place so you can be more *there where* you'd like to be, there where you *don't care* while the nurse *takes care* of the arm and the medicine. And, when it's over, then you'll be done, so when you're ready you can now return to your usual alertness and awareness".

K was also taught to use self-hypnosis to get rid of "those warts you don't need anymore". In each session, she experienced hypnosis so she could "use your imagination and creative mind to shrink yourself down in order to travel inside your body". She had already been taught about the blood vessels underneath the warts. The suggestion was given to "decide for yourself your own special way to stop the blood supply from feeding the warts". She heard a few ideas used by other children, such as a rope and lasso, a knife, a detour. Within a few moments her dominant handmade slashing gestures, as if she held a knife. Such ideomotor gestures are common during hypnosis.

K. practiced her self-hypnosis three times daily for two weeks, re-enacting the "scenes" elicited above. Upon return the warts were notably smaller, and she indicated readiness for the needed immunization. Two weeks later she returned again, wearing a lovely skirt, and proudly announced her successful experience with that immunization procedure. The warts were gone.

7.1.4. CASE #4: Adolescent with Chronic Daily Headache (HA)

W was 15-2/12 at the time of her first visit. She was referred by one of her two pediatric neurologists for help with chronic, daily, severe headaches.

A detailed history was taken, revealing headaches since early childhood that increased in frequency, duration, and severity over time. There was a very strong family history of migraines. Over the years, she was evaluated by many physicians at various clinics and hospitals for the continuing severe headaches triggered by "lack of sleep/water, MSG, scents, physical activity, thinking, breathing, living in general." Diagnostic testing for autonomic dysfunction revealed no positive results. Interventions included multiple medication trials, and a recent three-month intensive inpatient rehab program that involved a comprehensive and multi-modal approach: physical therapy, "group biofeedback", relaxation including diaphragmatic breathing, listening to music, meditation, progressive relaxation, distraction, socialization with games, reading, movies, peers and positive self-talk, and an agreement to avoid opioids and daily pain medications. There was no mention of hypnosis.

W.'s academic history was marked by absence and numerous changes in locations and types of schooling.

During the initial visit, the typical *assessment* scale to measure pain severity scale was also used *therapeutically*. Using an agreed upon range of 0–12 (12 = worst imaginable HA, 0 = none), her average was eight. Surprised with the question: "What would you *prefer*?" she replied, "Four or less but I don't think zero would be a good idea because I do feel I have this for a reason and it has enabled me to meet people." When asked the last time it was *zero* she indicated "before it became daily 17 months earlier".

The clinician gently corrected her by offering a *re-framing idea* that it is *zero* "whenever you are asleep" and in a purposely constructed "waking hypnotic suggestion", the clinician said "So, *all* we have to do really is find out how to move the file in your brain called *no headache* from only at night to also when you're awake". As with most patients with chronic recurrent pain, the clinician introduced the possibility of change while simultaneously assessing motivation through the use of embedded suggestions with carefully selected wording in the following questions:

Will you miss the HA's when they're gone? ➜ "No."

Is there anything good about the HA's? ➜ "No"

Do you need them for anything? ➜ "No"

Do you think you have had them long enough? ➜ "Yes"

Given W.'s very chronic and severe headache history without relief despite multiple interventions, the clinician then set a therapeutic goal to *shift her focus* from over-investment in her pain to positive expectations for self-healing. W. agreed to keep a written HA diary, and was given a therapeutic suggestion "to track the reduced frequency and intensity. The clinician also asked W. if she "needed to find or know the "reason" for the HA if she could find a way for it to not bother her", and she said she did NOT need to know the reason. *Of course had she said she did need to know the reason, additional and alternative clinical approaches would have been the appropriate next step.*

During the initial visit, multiple therapeutic seeds of "waking suggestions" were planted for her consideration, including (1) pain is pain, suffering is optional; (2) pain is a signal, nothing more, nothing less; and (3) when everything that can be done and should be done, has been done, there is no reason for pain to bother. At the end of this visit the clinician again evoked positive expectations when telling W. that he was absolutely sure he could *help her help herself*, that everyone whom he had ever met with a HA problem had gotten better without exception, and that she was invited to leave all past, present, and future headaches in the clinician's file cabinet. She laughed.

At the second visit, training in hypnosis and self hypnosis began with viewing a couple of videos of youngsters both talking about and doing self-hypnosis. Induction (initiation) of hypnosis was easily accomplished with "favorite place imagery". Suggestions for multisensory imagery along with progressive relaxation served to intensify (or "deepen") the hypnotic experience. To amplify that self-hypnosis training emphasizes personal choice and self-control, therapeutic hypnotic suggestions for controlling HA were offered as a "menu" from which W could choose. For example, she was told "I don't know how you will lower those HA's that used to be there more, but somewhere in your inner mind you know how because you want to be and can be the boss of those HA's instead of them begin the boss of you. I'd like to tell you some stories of how *other* young people got rid of *their* HA's….I knew this one 12-year-old boy who had migraines and he used the idea of being on an elevator, so if he had a migraine that was a '10', he'd push the button to ride down to nine, and then the light would go off at 10 and on at nine, and then eight….and then . . . . . . six or five . . . . . and . . . then . . . . all the way to one or zero," I met this one little girl who was only five; and she had a stomach-ache problem and she didn't like elevators, so what *she* did in *her* imagination was imagine being on a water slide; and the 12 was at the top and the zero was at the bottom in the cool refreshing water, and whenever she had a tummy ache she would get on the water slide in her mind and zooooommmm down from 11-10-9-8-7-6-5-4-3-2-1-splash! A few years ago, I worked with a 17-year-old young woman, with migraine problems, who rode horses. To control her migraines she'd imagine riding on the beach with the horses' hooves gradually erasing the zero–12 numbers in the sand. And, of course, when it got to zero it stayed there. I don't know which of those stories you'll use, or maybe some combination, or probably you've already come up with a couple in your own mind from your experiences. And, like everything, the more you practice, the better you'll get. Whichever works best for you is the best for you."

W. practiced self-hypnosis a couple of times each day as suggested. She improved gradually. She agreed to also keep a concurrent diary of "How am I dealing with it?" ratings, with zero = dealing with it best, and 12 = worst. W. soon reported much less use of medication for "severe" HA, and decrease of migraine prevention and anxiolytic medications.

By the middle of the following school year she was substantially improved. Nine months after the first visit, W. reported that her average HA rating was now down to 3.6 (from average of 8.5) and her "dealing with it" had improved 23%! to 2.3 With the intention of increasing her awareness of and empowering her own abilities the clinician asked W. "How did you DO that?" She replied "I am *stunned* it is *astonishing*... I never thought I could do it... you know, change my body with my mind. I did continue what you told me to do, so I imagine being at the cabin, and reading and then I swim in the lake and the closer I come back to shore the lower the number of my HA is and when I get to shore it's fine!"

8. Contraindications and Caveats

While the foregoing cases are representative of common conditions *and* common responses to hypnotic interventions, it is essential to note that not everyone responds so positively and so quickly. Like any strategic therapeutic intervention, positive rapport is essential to good clinical work, and ongoing re-evaluation, flexibility, and engagement in brainstorming with patients and families are fundamental to ultimate progress, problem resolution, and healing.

As with any clinical intervention, treatment with clinical hypnosis is not without obstacles or roadblocks. As with any skill, rehearsal ("practice") of self-hypnosis skills enhances competence, confidence, and positive outcomes whereas absence of regular rehearsal is more likely to result in slower and/or less positive results. We give "homework" assignments involving practice of self-hypnosis, counsel parents about their level of involvement *versus* interference, and encourage children and youth to come to appointments *with* their hypnosis and not only *for* it. Not unlike other therapies, however, inconsistent follow-up appointments and/or inconsistent attention to home rehearsal are potential contributors to less than desired outcomes.

For some children's problems—as noted in the foregoing tables, hypnosis may be clearly the treatment of choice (e.g., enuresis, migraine) and have the best "track record" compared to what might otherwise have been considered "traditional" approaches to that problem. By contrast, for other problems/conditions (e.g., behavioral and mental health issues) hypnosis may be clearly more adjunctive, but nonetheless highly valued as an important ingredient in an overall management plan (e.g., with asthma or other chronic illnesses where learning self-hypnosis may not provide "cure" or resolution, but can/will contribute to reduced morbidity such as less medication needs, fewer days missed from school, better sleep, *etc.*) [2,30].

9. Contraindications

There are a few absolute contraindications to the utilization of hypnosis with children, and several more relative contraindications [2].

- Hypnosis should not be utilized for entertainment. As we have discussed and illustrated, hypnosis is a very effective clinical tool; and often may have powerful and dramatic positive effects on medical and mental health. We strongly advocate against the use of hypnosis for public entertainment as is seen commonly during high school graduation parties.
- Hypnosis should only be used by clinicians trained in the appropriate use of hypnosis and hypnotherapy and within the scope of their clinical practice. Thus, while hypnosis/hypnotherapy are very appropriate and useful adjuncts to help children with anxiety and/or discomfort during dental work, it would of course be unethical and inappropriate for a pediatrician or a psychologist who has learned hypnosis to start doing dental extractions! Of course it would be appropriate for those professionals to teach their clients how to use self-hypnosis WHEN they go to the dentist).

Analogously, though hypnosis can be a very helpful tool in treating posttraumatic stress disorder (PTSD), clinicians who learn hypnosis yet have no specialized training in treating children with PTSD should not start offering hypnosis for PTSD.

- Hypnosis should not be used to treat a condition for which there is already a fundamentally appropriate, acceptable, accessible, and effective treatment. One example might be strep throat. Or appendicitis. Of course, however, one might well learn self-hypnosis to help allay anxiety or discomfort associated with having a throat culture; or learn methods of control of anxiety, discomfort, and return of normal bodily functions pre- and post-operatively for an appendectomy.
- Hypnosis should be tailored to the developmental level and capacities of the individual child. Designing a hypnosis session to address clinical anxiety for a six-year-old would be very different for a nine-year-old. Typically, developing toddlers and those children with significantly impaired intellectual and language abilities and limited capacity for internal absorption would benefit from repetitive sensorimotor stimuli known to induce a calmer, steadier state of comfort, such as rhythmic rocking, patting, swaying, or music.

10. HOW?: Learning Hypnosis Skills

While this article is intended to be an overview of the value of clinical hypnosis in children, it is neither a "HOW to do it…" nor a manual or a written suggestion to imply that clinicians reading this article can now go to the office and begin using hypnosis. Quite the contrary, even the case illustrations noted carry the **notable** *caveat* that the involved experienced pediatric clinicians were very well trained in pediatric clinical hypnosis *before* they began to apply these skills in their clinical work.

It is our hope and intention that the foregoing will serve as a stimulus for further study, inquiry, and most importantly, for appropriate clinical skill development through training by licensed health care professionals. Pediatric-specific didactic presentations and experiential learning through supervised practice by licensed pediatric professionals are essential to the development of the expertise required to help children and families help themselves through the learning of self-hypnosis in fostering self-regulation abilities and other internal resources, as well as symptom reduction.

As briefly noted earlier, starting in 1987, a cadre of multidisciplinary faculty of licensed health care professionals began teaching what has become the longest-running pediatric clinical hypnosis workshop training in the United States, sponsored by the Society for Developmental and Behavioral Pediatrics (SDBP). Beyond those twenty-four years of workshops, the enduring and growing Faculty initiated the National Pediatric Hypnosis Training Institute (NPHTI = nifty!) in 2010 which continues to provide the tri-level pediatric hypnosis training workshops annually. Over the past 4 years over 400 child health professionals with graduate degrees have availed themselves of the NPHTI skill development workshops. These past participants, representing over forty states in the U.S.A. and seven foreign countries, include pediatricians, pediatric subspecialists (e.g., developmental-behavioral pediatricians, pediatric-trained pulmonologists, gastroenterologists, neurologists, oncologists, anesthesiologists), pediatric psychologists and child and adolescent psychiatrists, pediatric social workers, marriage and family therapists, Child Life Specialists, advanced practice pediatric nurses (e.g., clinical nurse specialists, pediatric nurse practitioners, and advanced practice RNs), and pediatric occupational therapists and physical therapists.

NPHTI is a rapidly growing professional organization open to inquiries from licensed professionals with advanced degrees and would be pleased to welcome qualified applicants to future training. (See www.nphti.com).

Acknowledgments

We are grateful to our colleagues whose research and publications cited herein make this endeavor so exciting, and to the children and families with whom we are privileged to work and teach.

Author Contributions

Each author contributed two of the case reports, and contributed to, reviewed, and approved the text of the manuscript.

Conflicts of Interest

The authors declare no conflict of interest.

References

1. Mead, M. *Male and Female: A Study of the Sexes in a Changing World*; William Morrow: New York, NY, USA, 1949.
2. Kohen, D.P.; Olness, K.N. *Hypnosis and Hypnotherapy with Children*, 4th ed.; Routledge Publications, Taylor & Francis: New York, NY, USA, 2011.

3. Baldwin, J.M. Suggestion in Infancy. *Science* **1891**, *17*, 113–117.

4. Erickson, M.H. Pediatric Hypnotherapy. *Am. J. Clin. Hypn.* **1958**, *1*, 25–29.

5. Wright, M.E. Hypnosis and Child Therapy. *Am. J. Clin. Hypn.* **1960**, *2*, 197–205.

6. Baumann, F.W.; Hinman, F. Treatment of incontinent boys with non-obstructive disease. *J. Urol.* **1974**, *111*, 114–116.

7. Baumann, F.W. Hypnosis and the adolescent drug abuser. *Am. J. Clin. Hypn.* **1970**, *13*, 17–21.

8. London, P.; Cooper, L.M. Norms of hypnotic susceptibility in children. *Dev. Psychol.* **1969**, *1*, 113–124.

9. Barber, T.X.; Calverley, D.S. "Hypnotic-like" suggestibility in children. *J. Abnorm. Soc. Psychol.* **1963**, *66*, 589–597.

10. Gardner, G.G. Hypnotherapy in the management of childhood habit disorders. *J. Pediatr.* **1978**, *92*, 838–840.

11. Olness, K. The use of self-hypnosis in the treatment of childhood nocturnal enuresis. A report on forty patients. *Clin. Pediatr.* **1975**, *14*, 273–279.

12. Zeltzer, L.K.; LeBaron, S. Hypnosis and non-hypnotic techniques for reduction of pain and anxiety during painful procedures in children and adolescents with cancer. *J. Pediatr.* **1982**, *101*, 1032–1035.

13. Zeltzer, L.K.; LeBaron, S.; Zeltzer, P.M. The effectiveness of behavioral intervention for reducing nausea and vomiting in children and adolescents receiving chemotherapy. *J. Clin. Oncol.* **1984**, *2*, 683–690.

14. LeBaron, S.; Hilgard, J.R. *Hypnotherapy of Pain in Children with Cancer*; William Kaufman: Los Altos, CA, USA, 1984.

15. Olness, K.N. Case Western Reserve University, Cleveland, OH, USA. Personal Communication, 2014.

16. Gardner, G.G.; Olness, K.N. *Hypnosis and Hypnotherapy with Children*; Grune and Stratton: New York, NY, USA, 1981.

17. Olness, K.N.; Gardner, G.G. *Hypnosis and Hypnotherapy with Children*, 2nd ed; Guilford Press: New York, NY, USA, 1988.

18. Olness, K.N.; Kohen, D.P. *Hypnosis and Hypnotherapy with Children*; Guilford Press: New York, NY, USA, 1996.

19. Olness K.N.; Kohen, D.P. Lehrbuch der Kinderhypnose und hypnotherapie; Carl-Auer-Systeme Verlag, 2001. (originally published in English under the title Hypnosis and Hypnotherapy with Children, 3rd ed.; The Guilford Press: New York, NY, USA, 1996. see reference 18 above).

20. Olness, K.; Kohen, D.P. Hypnose et Hypnotherapie chez l'enfant; SATAS s.a.: Bruxelles, Belgiques, 2006. (Original: Hypnosis and Hypnotherapy with Children; Olness, K., Kohen, D.P., Eds.; Guilford Press: New York, NY, USA, 1996, see reference 18 above).

21. Kohen, D.P.; Olness, K.N.; Colwell, S.; Heimel, A. The use of relaxation/mental imagery (self-hypnosis) in the management of 505 pediatric behavioral encounters. *J. Dev. Behav. Pediatr.* **1984**, *1*, 21–25.

22. Kuttner, L. No Fears, No Tears (29 min). DVD available online: http://bookstore.cw.bc.ca (accessed on 15 May 2014).

23. Kuttner, L. No Fears, No Tears 13 Years Later: Children Coping with Pain (46 min). DVD available online: http://bookstore.cw.bc.ca (accessed on 15 May 2014).

24. Kuttner, L. Favourite stories. A hypnotic pain reduction technique for children in acute pain. *Am. J. Clin. Hypn.* **1988**, *30*, 289–295.

25. Kuttner, L. *Making Every Moment Count Documentary* (38 min); Co-production with The National Film Board of Canada, 2003. Available online: www.nfb.ca (accessed on 15 May 2014).

26. Olness, K.N.; Culbert, T.C.; Uden, D. Self-regulation of salivary immunoglobulin A by children. *Pediatrics* **1989**, *83*, 66–71.

27. Sugarman, L.I. *Hypnosis in Pediatric Practice: Imaginative Medicine in Action*; DVD and booklet; Crown House Publishing: Carmarthen, Wales, UK, 2006.

28. Thomson, L. *Harry Hypno-Potamus: Metaphorical Tales for Pediatric Problems*; Crown House Publishing Bancyfelin: Carmarthen, UK, 2005.

29. Thomson, L. *Harry Hypno-Potamus: More Metaphorical Tales for Pediatric Problems*; Crown House Publishing: Bancyfelin, Carmarthen, UK, 2009; Volume 2.

30. Sugarman, L.I.; Wester, W.C. *Therapeutic Hypnosis with Children and Adolescents*, 2nd ed; Crown House Publishing: Bancyfelin Carmarthen, Wales, UK, 2014.

31. National Pediatric Hypnosis Training Institute. Available online: www.nphti.com (accessed on 20 May 2014).

32. Trenkle, B. Kindertagung History—Heidelberg, Germany. Personal Communication, May 2014. Available online: http://www.trenkle-organisation.de (accessed on 21 May 2014).

33. Kohen, D.P. Relaxation/Mental imagery (self-hypnosis) for childhood asthma: Behavioral outcomes in a prospective, controlled study. *Hypnos* **1995**, *22*, 132–143.

34. Kohen, D.P.; Wynne, E. Applying hypnosis in a preschool family asthma education program: Uses of storytelling, imagery and relaxation. *Am. J. Clin. Hypn.* **1997**, *39*, 2–14.

35. Kohen, D.P.; Botts P. Relaxation-imagery (self-hypnosis) in Tourette syndrome: Experience with four children. *Am. J. Clin. Hypn.* **1987**, *29*, 227–237.

36. Lynn, S.J.; Rhue, J.W. *Theories of Hypnosis: Current Models and Perspectives*; Guilford Press: New York, NY, USA, 1991.

37. The Society of Psychological Hypnosis, Division 30 of the American Psychological Association. Available online: http://psychologicalhypnosis.com/info/ (accessed on 5 May 2014).

38. Sugarman, L.I. Re-Thinking Hypnosis/Refining Utilization. In Proceedings of Intermediate Pediatric Hypnosis Workshop—National Pediatric Hypnosis Training Institute, Minneapolis, MN, USA, 3 October 2013.

39. Rainville, P.; Carrier, B.; Hoffbauer, R.K.; Bushnell, M.C.; Duncan, G.H. Dissociation of sensory and affective dimensions of pain using hypnotic modulation. *Pain* **2001**, *82*, 159–171.

40. Raz, A. Does neuroimaging of suggestion elucidate hypnotic trance? *Int. J. Clin. Exp. Hypn.* **2011**, *59*, 363–377.

41. Wagstaff, G.F. On the centrality of the concept of an altered state to definitions of hypnosis. *J. Mind-Body Regul.* **2014**, *2*, 90–108.

42. Kaiser, P. Chlldhood Anxiety, Worry, and Fear: Individualizing Hypnosis Goals and Suggestions for Self-Regulation. *Am. J. Clin. Hypn.* **2011**, *54*, 16–31.

43. Berger, A. *Self-Regulation: Brain, Cognition, and Development*; American Psychological Association: Washington, DC, USA, 2011.

44. Hall, H. Resources for Future Training. Presented at National Pediatric Hypnosis Training Institute Introductory Workshop, Chaska, MN, USA, 5 October 2013.

45. Kohen, D.P. A pediatric perspective on mind-body medicine. In *Integrative Pediatrics*; Culbert, T.P., Olness, K., Eds.; Oxford University Press: New York, NY, USA, 2010; pp. 267–301.

46. Yapko, M.D. *Trancework: An Introduction to the Practice of Clinical Hypnosis*, 4th ed.; Routledge: New York, NY, USA, 2012.

47. Benson, H. *The Relaxation Response*, 2nd ed.; Avon Books: New York, NY, USA, 1990.

48. Kohen, D.P. Interview and demonstration of Relaxation and Mental Imagery for an 11 y.o. Boy (John H.) with Asthma and Anxiety, Minneapolis, MN, USA, 1996.

49. Olness, K.; MacDonald, J.T.; Uden, D.L. Comparison of self-hypnosis and propranolol in the treatment of juvenile classic migraine. *Pediatrics* **1987**, *79*, 593–597.

50. Dikel, W.; Olness, K. Self-hypnosis, biofeedback, and voluntary peripheral temperature control in children. *Pediatrics* **1980**, *66*, 335–340.

51. Olness, K.N.; Conroy, M. Voluntary control of transcutaneous pO2 by children. *Int. J. Clin. Exp. Hypn.* **1985**, *33*, 1–5.

52. Kohen, D.P.; Ondich, S. Children's self-regulation of cardiovascular function with relaxation mental imagery (self-hypnosis): Report of a controlled study. *Hypnos: J. Eur. Soc. Hypn. Psychother. Psychosom. Med.* **2004**, *31*, 61–74.

53. Lee, L.H.; Olness, K.N. Effects of self-induced mental imagery on autonomic reactivity in children. *J. Dev. Behav. Pediatr.* **1996**, *17*, 323–327.

54. Anbar, R.D. Self-hypnosis for patients with cystic fibrosis. *Pediatr. Pulm.* **2000**, *30*, 461–465.

55. Olness, K.N. Imagery (self-hypnosis) as adjunctive therapy in childhood cancer: Clinical experience with 25 patients. *Am. J. Pediatr. Hem./Onc.* **1981**, *3*, 313–321.

56. Jacknow, D.S.; Tschann, J.M.; Link, M.P.; Boyce, W.T. Hypnosis in the prevention of chemotherapy—Related nausea and vomiting in children: A prospective study. *J. Dev. Behav. Pediatr.* **1994**, *15*, 22–306.

57. Kohen, D.P.; Zajac, R. Self-hypnosis training for headaches in children and adolescents. *J. Pediatr.* **2007**, *150*, 635–639.

58. Kohen, D.P. Long-term follow-up of self-hypnosis training for recurrent headaches: What the children say. *Int. J. Clin. Exp. Hypn.* **2010**, *58*, 417–432.

59. Sugarman, L.I.; Garrison, B.L.; Williford, K.L. Symptoms as solutions: Hypnosis and biofeedback for autonomic regulation in autism spectrum disorders. *Am. J. Clin. Hypn.* **2013**, *56*, 152–173.

60. Kohen, D.P. Management of trichotillomania with relaxation/mental imagery (self-hypnosis): Experience with five children. *J. Dev. Behav. Pediatr.* **1996**, *17*, 328–334.

61. Thomson, L. Hypnosis for habit disorders. Helping children help themselves. *Adv. Nurse Pract.* **2002**, *10*, 59–62.

62. Gottsegen, D.N. Curing bedwetting on the spot: A review of one session cures. *Clin. Pediatr. (Phila)* **2003**, *42*, 273–275.

63. Anbar, R.D.; Hall, H.R. Childhood habit cough treated with self-hypnosis. *J. Pediatr.* **2004**, *144*, 213–217.

64. Shenefelt, P.D. Using hypnosis to facilitate resolution of psychogenic excoriations in acne excoriee. *Am. J. Clin. Hypn.* **2004**, *46*, 239–245.

65. Anbar, R.D. User friendly hypnosis as an adjunct for treatment of habit cough: A case report. *Am. J. Clin. Hypn.* **2007**, *50*, 171–175.

66. Cyr, L.R.; Culbert, T.; Kaiser, P. Helping children with stress and anxiety: An integrative medicine approach. *Biofeedback* **2003**, *31*, 12–17.

67. Tschann, J.; Kaiser, P.; Boyce, W.T.; Chesney, M.A.; Alkon-Leonard, A. Resilience and vulnerability among preschoolers: Family functioning, temperament, and behavior problems. *J. Child Adol. Psychiatry* **1996**, *35*, 184–192.

68. Culbert, T.; Richtsmeier-Cyr, L. Pediatric Mind/Body Medicine: The Hypnosis/ Biofeedback Interface. (Entire Issue). In *Biofeedback Newsmagazine of the AAPB*; Culbert, T., Richtsmeier-Cyr, L., Eds.; The Association for Applied Psychophysiology and Biofeedback (AAPB): Wheat Ridge, CO, USA, 2005.

69. Olness, K. Self control and regulation. In *Developmental Behavioral Pediatrics*, 4th ed.; Carey, W., Crocker, A., Elias, E., Feldman, H., Coleman, W., Eds.; Saunders: Philadelphia, PA, USA, 2009.

70. Yapko, M. *Mindfulness and Hypnosis: The Power of Suggestion to Transform Experience*; W.W. Norton & Co.: New York, NY, USA, 2011.

71. Kohen, D.P. Chronic daily headache: Helping adolescents help themselves with self-hypnosis. *Am. J. Clin. Hypn.* **2011**, *54*, 32–46.

72. Labaw, W.L. Auto-hypnosis in hemophilia. *Haematologia* **1975**, *9*, 103–110.

73. Anbar, R.D. Self-hypnosis for anxiety associated with severe asthma: A case report. *BMC Pediatr.* **2003**, *3*, 7.

74. Hackman, R.M.; Stern, J.S.; Gershwin, M.E. Hypnosis and asthma: A critical review. *J. Asthma.* **2000**, *b37*, 1–15.

75. Culbert, T.; Kajander, R.; Kohen, D.; Reaney, J. Hypnobehavioral approaches for school-age children with dysphagia and food aversion. *J. Dev. Behav. Pediatr.* **1996**, *17*, 335–341.

76. Gottsegen, D. Hypnosis for functional abdominal pain. *Am. J. Clin. Hypn.* **2011**, *54*, 56–69.

77. Kuttner, L.; Chambers, C.T.; Hardial, J.; Israel, D.M.; Jacobsen, K.; Evans, K. A randomized trial of yoga for adolescents with irritable bowel syndrome. *Pain Res. Manag.* **2006**, *11*, 217–223.

78. Vlieger, A.M.; Menko-Frankenhuis, C.; Wolfkamp, S.C.S. Hypnotherapy for children with functional abdominal pain or Irritable Bowel Syndrome: A randomized controlled trial. *Gastroenterology* **2007**, *133*, 1430–1436.

79. Pendergrast, R.A. Imagine Something Different. *Arch. Pediatr. Adolesc. Med.* **2003**, *157*, 325–326.

80. Kohen, D.P. Ericksonian communication and hypnotic strategies in the management of tics and Tourette syndrome in children and adolescents with Tourette syndrome. In *Difficult Contexts for Therapy—Ericksonian Monographs*; Lankton, S.R., Zeig, J.K., Eds.; Brunner/Mazel: New York, NY, USA, 1995; Volume 10, pp. 117–142.

81. Kuttner, L. Pain—An integrative approach. In *Oxford Textbook of Palliative Care for Children*; Goldman, A., Hain, R., Liben, S., Eds.; Oxford University Press: New York, NY, USA, 2006; pp. 332–341.

82. Berberich, F.R.; Landman, Z. Reducing immunization discomfort in 4- to 6-year-old children: A randomized clinical trial. *Pediatrics* **2009**, *124*, e203–e209.

83. Myers, C.D.; Bergman, J.; Zeltzer, L.K. Complementary and alternative medicine use in children with cancer. In *Psychosocial Aspects of Pediatric Oncology*; Kreitler, S., Arush, M.B., Eds.; John Wiley and Sons: Hoboken, NJ, USA, 2004; pp. 335–350.

84. Zeltzer, L.K.; Dolgin, M.J.; LeBaron, S.; LeBaron, C. A randomized, controlled study of behavioral intervention for chemotherapy distress in children with cancer. *Pediatrics* **1991**, *88*, 34–42.

85. Anbar, R.D. Self-hypnosis for management of chronic dyspnea in pediatric patients. *Pediatrics* **2001**, *107*, 395–396.

86. Antich, J.L.S. The use of hypnosis in pediatric anesthesia. *J. Am. Soc. Psychosom. Dent. Med.* **1967**, *14*, 70–73.

87. Bernstein, N.R. Observations on the use of hypnosis with burned children on a pediatric ward. *Int. J. Clin. Exp. Hypn.* **1965**, *13*, 1–10.

88. Butler, L.D.; Symons, B.K.; Henderson, S.L.; Shortliffe, L.D.; Spiegel, D. Hypnosis Reduces Distress and Duration of an Invasive Medical Procedure for Children. *Pediatrics* **2005**, *115*, 77–85.

89. French, G.M.; Painter, E.C.; Coury, D.L. Blowing away shot pain: A technique for pain management during immunization. *Pediatrics* **1994**, *93*, 384–390.

90. Kohen, D.P. Applications of relaxation/mental imagery (self-hypnosis) in pediatric emergencies. *Int. J. Clin. Exp. Hypn.* **1996**, *34*, 283–294.

91. Kuttner, L. *A Child in Pain: How to Help: What Health Professionals Can Do to Help Crown*; House Publishing: Bethel, CT, USA, 2010.

92. Tsao, J.C.I.; Meldrum, M.; Kim, S.C.; Jacob, M.C. Treatment preferences for CAM in pediatric chronic pain patients. *Evid.-Based Complement. Altern. Med.* **2007**, *4*, 367–374.

93. Uman, L.S.; Chambers, C.T.; McGrath, P.J.; Kisely, S.A. A systematic review of randomized controlled trials examining psychological interventions for needle-related procedural pain and distress in children and adolescents: An abbreviated Cochrane Review. *J. Pediatr. Psychol.* **2008**, *33*, 842–854.

94. Kaiser, P. Childhood anxiety and psychophysiological reactivity: Hypnosis to build discrimination and self-regulation skills. *Am. J. Clin. Hypn.* **2014**, *56*, 343–367.

152

95. Spies, G. Desensitization of test anxiety: Hypnosis compared with biofeedback. *Am. J. Clin. Hypn.* **1979**, *22*, 108–111.

96. Kuttner, L.; Friedrichsdorf, S.J. *Hypnosis and palliative care In Therapeutic Hypnosis with Children and Adolescents*, 2nd ed.; Sugarman, L.I., Wester, W.C., II, Eds.; Crown House Publishing: Bancyfelin, Carmarthen, Wales, UK, 2014; pp. 491–509.

97. Golden, W. Cognitive Hypnotherapy for Anxiety Disorders. *Am. J. Clin. Hypn.* **2012**, *54*, 263–274.

98. Kerns, C.M.; Read, K.L.; Klugman, J.; Kendall, P.C. Cognitive-behavioral therapy for youth with social anxiety: Differential short and long-term treatment outcomes. *J. Anxiety Disord.* **2013**, *27*, 210–215.

99. Yapko, M.D. *Treating Depression With Hypnosis: Integrating Cognitive-Behavioral and Strategic Approaches*; Brunner-Routledge: New York, NY, USA, 2001.

100. Yapko, M.D. *Applying Hypnosis in Treating Depression: Innovations in Clinical Practice*; Routledge Press: New York, NY, USA, 2006.

101. Kohen, D.P.; Murray, K. Depression in Children and Youth: Applications of Hypnosis to Help Young People Help Themselves. In *Applying Hypnosis in Treating Depression: Innovations in Clinical Practice*; Yapko, M.D., Ed.; Routledge Press: New York, NY, USA, 2006; pp. 189–216.

102. Kohen, D.P. Depression. In *Therapeutic Hypnosis with Children and Adolescents*; Sugarman, L.I., Wester, W.C., II, Eds.; Crown House Publishing: Bancyfelin, Carmarthen, Wales, UK, 2014; Chapter 9, pp. 187–208.

103. Culbert, T.; Kajander, R. *Be the Boss of Your Sleep: Self-Care for Kids*; FreeSpirit Press: Minneapolis, MN, USA, 2007.

104. Kuttner, L. Treating pain, anxiety and sleep disorders with children and adolescents. In *Advances in the Use of Hypnosis in Medicine, Dentistry, Pain Prevention and Management*; Brown, D.C., Ed.; Crown House Publishers: Bethel, CT, USA, 2009; Chapter 11, pp. 177–194.

105. Kohen, D.P.; Mahowald, M.W.; Rosen, G.R. Sleep-terror disorder in children: The role of self-hypnosis in management. *Am. J. Clin. Hypn.* **1992**, *34*, 233–244.

106. Stanton, H.E.: Hypnotic relaxation and the reduction of sleep onset insomnia. *Int. J. Psychosom.* **1989**, *36*, 64–68.

107. Zeltzer, L.K.; Schlank, C. *Conquering your Child's Chronic Pain*; Harper and Collins: New York, NY, USA, 2005.

108. Gardner, G.G. Childhood, death and human dignity: Hypnotherapy for David. *Int J. Clin. Exp. Hypn.* **1976**, *24*, 122–139.

109. Gulewitsch, M.; Muller, J.; Hautzinger, M.; Schlarb, A.A. Brief hypnotherapeutic-behavioral intervention for functional abdominal pain and irritable bowel syndrome in childhood: A randomized controlled trial. *Eur. J. Pediatr.* **2013**, *172*, 1043–1051.

110. Schlarb, A.A.; Liddle, C.C.; Hautzinger, M. JuSt—A multimodal treatment program for adolescents with insomnia. Pilot study. *Nat. Sci. Sleep.* **2011**, *3*, 13–20.

111. Lifshitz, M.; Cusumano, E.P.; Raz, A. Hypnosis as neurophenomenology. *Front. Hum. Neurosci.* **2013**, doi:10.3389/fnhum.2013.00469.

112. Curtis, S.; Wingert, A.; Ali, S. *The Cochrane Library* and Procedural Pain in Children: An Overview of Reviews. *Evid.-Based Child Health: A Cochrane Rev. J.* **2012**, *7*, 1363–1399. doi:10.1002/ebch.1864.

113. Gold, J.I.; Kant, A.J.; Belmont, K.A.; Butler, L.D. Practitioner review: Clinical applications of pediatric hypnosis. *J. Child Psychol. Psychiatry* **2007**, *48*, 744–754.

114. Landier, W.; Tse, A. Use of Complementary and Alternative Medical Interventions for the Managaement of Procedure-Related Pain, Anxiety, and Distress in Pediatric Oncology: An Integrative Review. *J. Pediatr. Nurs.* **2010**, *25*, 566–579.

115. McClafferty, H. Complementary, Holistic, and Integrative Medicine: Mind-Body Medicine. *Pediatr. Rev.* **2011**, *32*, 201–203.

116. Richardson, J.; Smith, J.; McCall, G.; Pilkington, J. Hypnosis for Procedure-Related Pain and Distress in Pediatric Cancer Patients: A Systematic Review of Effectiveness and Methodology Related to Hypnosis Interventions. *J. Pain Symp. Manag.* **2006**, *31*, 70–84.

117. Schnur, J.B.; Kafer, I.; Marcus, C.; Montgomery, G.H. Hypnosis to Manage Distress Related to Medical Procedures: A Meta-Analysis. *Contemp Hypn.* **2008**, *25*, 114–128, doi:10.1002/ch.364.

118. Uman, L.S.; Birnie, K.A.; Noel, M.; Parker, J.A.; Chambers, C.T.; McGrath, P.J.; Kisely, S.R. Psychological interventions for needle-related procedural pain and distress in children and adolescents. *Cochrane Database Syst. Rev.* **2013**, *10*, doi:10.1002/14651858.CD005179.pub3.

Pediatric Integrative Medicine in Residency (PIMR): Description of a New Online Educational Curriculum

Hilary McClafferty, Sally Dodds, Audrey J. Brooks, Michelle G. Brenner, Melanie L. Brown, Paige Frazer, John D. Mark, Joy A. Weydert, Graciela M. G. Wilcox, Patricia Lebensohn and Victoria Maizes

Abstract: Use of integrative medicine (IM) is prevalent in children, yet availability of training opportunities is limited. The Pediatric Integrative Medicine in Residency (PIMR) program was designed to address this training gap. The PIMR program is a 100-hour online educational curriculum, modeled on the successful Integrative Medicine in Residency program in family medicine. Preliminary data on site characteristics, resident experience with and interest in IM, and residents' self-assessments of perceived knowledge and skills in IM are presented. The embedded multimodal evaluation is described. Less than one-third of residents had IM coursework in medical school or personal experience with IM. Yet most (66%) were interested in learning IM, and 71% were interested in applying IM after graduation. Less than half of the residents endorsed pre-existing IM knowledge/skills. Average score on IM medical knowledge exam was 51%. Sites endorsed 1–8 of 11 site characteristics, with most (80%) indicating they had an IM practitioner onsite and IM trained faculty. Preliminary results indicate that the PIMR online curriculum targets identified knowledge gaps. Residents had minimal prior IM exposure, yet expressed strong interest in IM education. PIMR training site surveys identified both strengths and areas needing further development to support successful PIMR program implementation.

Reprinted from *Children*. Cite as: McClafferty, H.; Dodds, S.; Brooks, A.J.; Brenner, M.G.; Brown, M.L.; Frazer, P.; Mark, J.D.; Weydert, J.A.; Wilcox, G.M.G.; Lebensohn, P.; *et al*. Pediatric Integrative Medicine in Residency (PIMR): Description of a New Online Educational Curriculum. *Children* **2015**, *2*, 98-107.

1. Introduction

Integrative medicine (IM) is prevention-based medicine that emphasizes the therapeutic patient-clinician relationship and uses all appropriate therapies [1]. IM has unique potential in pediatrics, where acquisition of healthy habits may confer lifelong benefits.

The integrative approach is personalized and addresses nutrition, mind-body medicine, sleep, exercise, whole medical systems (e.g., traditional Chinese medicine), environmental health, and social support.

Interest in IM is significant, driven by consumer demand for care that is cost effective and better aligned with patient values [2,3]. A 2005 Institute of Medicine statement recommended that health professional schools include education on complementary medicine at all training levels [4], highlighting the need for physician education. Guidelines on IM education have been published for medical students and family medicine residents [5–7]. Fellowship competencies exist for IM [8], and Board certification is now available for physicians [9].

Training in IM occurred quickly in some specialties. A four-year combined residency and fellowship in family medicine and integrative medicine launched in 2004 [10]. A 200-hour online IM curriculum (Integrative Medicine in Residency, IMR) developed in 2008 [11] is now used by more than 900 residents and 50 faculty members at 42 residencies.

Pediatrics lacks IM training programs, despite data from the 2007 National Health Interview Survey demonstrating that nearly 12% of all children used complementary therapies, with prevalence increasing to 50% in those with chronic illnesses [12]. Pediatricians' desire for education about complementary therapies was documented in an American Academy of Pediatrics (AAP) members' survey (n = 733) [2,13].

Despite significant IM use in children and interest among pediatricians, only 16 of 143 pediatric academic programs surveyed reported having IM programs in 2012 [3]. This gap presented an opportunity to design, implement, and evaluate a pilot program (Pediatric Integrative Medicine in Residency, PIMR). Alignment of the curriculum with newly developed Accreditation Council for Graduate Medical Education (ACGME) core competencies facilitated introduction of material on empathy, self-regulation skills, and the importance of self-care in residency training [14].

This article describes the PIMR program, a 100-hour online curriculum developed at the Arizona Center for Integrative Medicine (AzCIM) at the University of Arizona, currently being implemented at five residencies. Successful implementation will rely on a program's capacity to adopt new curriculum, and on resident readiness to learn about IM. Therefore, data will be presented on residency site characteristics, resident experience with and interest in IM, and residents' self-assessments of perceived IM knowledge and skills.

2. Methods

2.1. Curriculum Development

Content development was based on: guidelines from the joint ACGME and American Board of Pediatrics (ABP) "Pediatric Milestone Project" [15]; competencies in IM [8]; literature review of pediatric IM topics; and input from nationally recognized pediatric faculty. The curriculum provides: (1) an introduction to pediatric IM; (2) a review of foundational topics; and (3) case-based IM management of common conditions. Content was piloted at the University of Arizona pediatric residency then refined based on faculty and resident feedback and a needs assessment questionnaire distributed to faculty and residents at two academic pediatric training programs. Refinements included emphasis on self-care, case-based learning, and intake and treatment planning. Authors were fellowship-trained integrative pediatricians. Table 1 summarizes the curriculum.

The online curriculum is modular. Self-contained units can be adapted for use in core rotations, used within electives, or distributed longitudinally. Interactivity is facilitated with case-based teaching. Onsite teaching and experiential activities tailored by the faculty site leaders round out the program. Onsite activities may include case conferences, self-care assessments, and experiential seminars. An annual faculty retreat provides faculty support and maintenance of current IM training.

The PIMR program's website is the hub of the resident learning community and includes online dialogues for questions and comments. Faculty site leaders track resident participation and course

156

completion through an online dashboard. Faculty resources are housed on the PIMR website and include an article archive, intake forms, handouts, and patient education materials. Linked access is provided to the Natural Medicines Database.

Evaluation of the PIMR program's curriculum is embedded into the website, organized into four components: (1) medical knowledge test and self-assessment; (2) course completion rates; (3) curriculum evaluation; and, (4) assessment of resident wellbeing and wellness behaviors. Both quantitative and qualitative methods are used. The University of Arizona Institutional Review Board (IRB) approved the study, as did required pilot site IRBs.

Table 1. Pediatric Integrative Medicine in Residency (PIMR) curriculum content.

Core Content	No. Hours
Introduction to Integrative Medicine	3
Introduction to Integrative Medicine	1
Medical Informatics	2
Self-Care	7
Introduction to Self-Care	1
Burnout & Stress	1
Mindfulness in Medicine	1
The Anti-Inflammatory Diet	2
Exercise & Sleep	1
Self-Care Wrap-up	1
Mind-Body	14
Introduction to Integrative Mental Health	6
Spirituality & Health Care	2
Mind-Body Medicine in Practice	6
Nutrition & Physical Activity	12
Nutrition Fundamentals	6
Nutrition Case Studies	5
Physical Activity for Children	1
Dietary Supplements	19
Micronutrients & Supplements: An Introduction	1
Vitamins & Minerals	7.5
Common Dietary Supplements	6.5
Botanical Foundations	4
Whole Systems	13
Whole Systems Introduction	5
Manual Medicine	8
Clinical Focus	32
Motivational Interviewing	3
Integrative Intake & Treatment Plan	3
Integrative Pediatric Neurology	5
Environmental Medicine: An Integrative Approach	6
Immunizations	1
Integrative Dermatology	4
Integrative Respiratory Health	10
TOTAL HOURS	100

2.2. Pilot Sites and Selection

In 2012, five residency programs were selected to participate in a three-year project to implement and evaluate the PIMR program's curriculum. Site inclusion criteria included endorsement by the Department Chair and Residency Director, and agreement to deliver the entire 100-hour curriculum to all residents over three years. Pilot sites include four university affiliated or based residencies and one community hospital residency. Sites vary in annual class size from 9 to 28 residents.

2.3. Measures

The following measures were used to assess program capacity to implement the curriculum and resident interest and readiness to learn about IM:

A. Site Capacity to Implement the PIMR Program: Pilot Site Characteristics. Within the first year of the PIMR program's implementation, program leaders at each site completed an 11-item checklist assessing infrastructure characteristics supportive of PIMR implementation. Characteristics include an established IM culture, faculty background in IM, and site activities supporting the PIMR curriculum.

B. Resident Interest in and Readiness for IM Training. Resident interest in and readiness for learning IM was assessed with three measures: (1) An eight-item *post-match survey* assessing prior IM/CAM (complementary alternative medicine) medical school coursework, personal use of IM/CAM, interest in learning IM, and interest in applying IM upon graduation. Items concerning prior IM experience were rated dichotomously (yes/no). Interest in learning and applying IM were rated on a 5-point scale; (2) A 32-item *resident self-assessment questionnaire* measuring confidence with IM knowledge and practice skills and ability to provide an IM approach to specific medical conditions. Items were rated on a 5-point scale from strongly disagree to strongly agree; and, (3) A 49-item *medical knowledge test* based on course content.

3. Results and Discussion

3.1. A. Site Capacity to Implement the PIMR Program: Pilot Site Characteristics

Four of five sites had the two most commonly found site readiness characteristics: an IM practitioner working onsite (IM culture), and faculty with IM training and resources. Sites varied in overall capacity to implement the PIMR program, ranging from endorsing only 1 characteristic (site E) to endorsing 8 (of the possible 11) characteristics (site C). See Table 2.

3.2. B. Resident Interest in and Readiness for IM Training

Sample. Of the 107 incoming class of 2016 residents, 97 completed the post-match, self-assessment, and/or medical knowledge measures (91% response rate). Of these, 75% were female, 68% were Caucasian, and 5% were Hispanic. Most were US medical school graduates (77%), 7% were osteopathic medical school graduates, and 16% were foreign medical school graduates.

Post-match Survey. The survey was completed prior to the July 1 start date. Less than one-third had IM/CAM coursework in medical school or personal experience with IM/CAM modalities. Sixty-six percent were interested in learning IM and 71% indicated interest in applying IM after graduation. See Table 3.

Table 2. Site characteristics by PIMR pilot site—baseline assessment.

Site	Site A	Site B	Site C	Site D	Site E	# Sites	% Sites
Faculty practicing IM consultation in the residency			X	X		2	40%
IM consultation available on site			X	X		2	40%
Other practitioners working on site	X	X	X	X		4	80%
MD and DO accredited residency, with osteopathic manipulation teaching on site		X				1	20%
IM fellowship available			X		X	2	40%
IM Culture Site Total	1	2	4	3	1	N/A	N/A
Faculty leader fellowship trained?	X	X	X	X		4	80%
Faculty leader with designated time to work on IM teaching	X	X	X	X		4	80%
Faculty Characteristics Site Total	2	2	2	2	0	N/A	N/A
Other IM teaching, rotation (1 month, 1–2 weeks), IM electives			X	X		2	40%
Case conferences monthly						0	0%
IM Retreats						0	0%
Support for residents applying knowledge in the clinic			X	X		2	40%
Additional IM Activities Site Total	0	0	2	2	0	N/A	N/A

Table 3. Postmatch survey results—N = 95 responding.

Item	N Percent	Mean ±SD
IM/CAM Experience		
Required IM/CAM coursework in medical school—N/% Yes	28.7%	N/A
IM/CAM electives in medical school—N/% Yes	25.5%	N/A
Personal Use of IM/CAM therapies or visits with IM/CAM providers—N/% Yes	30.9%	N/A
Interest in IM in Residency/Practice		
Interest in learning IM in residency—N/% Interested/Very Interested	66.0%	3.7 ± 1.2
Interest in applying IM in practice after residency—N/% Interested/Very Interested	71.3%	3.7 ± 1.2

Self-Assessment. The highest rated knowledge/skills items concerned: patient behavior change, familiarity with diets targeting cardiovascular disease, and physical activity recommendations. The lowest rated knowledge/skills items concerned dietary supplements and whole systems medicine. The ability to apply an integrative approach to medical conditions was highest for sleep, depression, and migraines, and lowest for rheumatoid arthritis, hyperlipidemia, and Type II Diabetes. See Table 4.

Table 4. Self-assessment of IM knowledge and skills/applying IM approach to medical conditions—means, standard deviations, and percent endorsing *(Items are presented from highest to lowest mean rating)* N = 91.

Item	Mean	SD	% Agree/ Strongly Agree
Knowledge/Skills			
I know how to assess a patient's readiness to change behavior.	3.31	0.77	48.6%
I know how to facilitate a patient's efforts at changing behaviors.	3.22	0.75	45.0%
I know the fundamental components of the Mediterranean and DASH diets as they relate to reduce risk of cardiovascular disease.	3.12	1.03	40.4%
I am aware of the different physical activity recommendations for children and adolescents.	3.03	0.84	38.5%
I can identify areas in my clinical setting that could be enhanced to promote wellbeing and healing.	2.93	1.07	35.8%
I know what the fundamental tenets of Integrative Medicine are.	2.56	0.86	16.5%
I feel competent in identifying nutritional needs based on gender, age and special populations for health promotion and disease prevention.	2.56	0.84	19.3%
I know how to take a spiritual history.	2.41	0.85	14.7%
I know the science of different mind-body techniques such as meditation, mindfulness, guided imagery, and biofeedback.	2.34	0.91	12.8%
I can identify the similarities and differences among the manual medicine modalities of massage, physical therapy, osteopathy and chiropractic.	2.33	0.97	14.7%
I can make recommendations in a patient-centered manner about an integrative treatment plan.	2.27	0.82	11.0%
I can identify the different components of an integrative treatment plan.	2.24	0.77	9.2%
I can identify the elements of an Integrative Patient intake.	2.23	0.79	7.3%
I know how to engage patients to assess mind-body interactions and their effects on health and wellness.	2.22	0.83	10.1%
I know the different theoretical and philosophical principles of Traditional Chinese Medicine (TCM), Ayurvedic Medicine, homeopathy, and Naturopathy.	1.91	0.92	7.3%
I know how to interpret the labels on herbal medicines.	1.89	0.83	4.6%
I can identify authoritative sources about botanicals.	1.87	0.80	4.6%
I know how to recommend botanicals to patients appropriately and safely.	1.67	0.67	0.9%
Medical Conditions			
Sleep disorders	2.70	1.04	28.4%
Depression	2.69	1.05	26.9%
Migraine Headaches	2.54	1.02	26.6%
Obesity	2.47	0.93	19.4%
Allergies	2.43	0.94	20.2%
Menstrual disorders	2.38	0.98	15.6%
ADHD	2.37	0.97	20.4%

Table 4. *Cont.*

Item	Mean	SD	% Agree/ Strongly Agree
Irritable Bowel Syndrome	2.37	1.01	15.6%
Asthma	2.34	0.90	12.8%
Eating Disorder	2.32	0.90	11.0%
Metabolic Syndrome	2.31	0.91	12.8%
Diabetes Mellitus type II	2.30	0.91	13.8%
Hyperlipidemia	2.30	0.91	13.8%
Rheumatoid arthritis	2.19	0.86	9.2%

Medical Knowledge. The average medical knowledge score was 51.3%, ranging from 35% to 78% (n = 76).

4. Discussion

Integrative medicine offers a powerful approach to a healthy lifestyle and can expand treatment options in children and adolescents. Use of complementary therapies is high in children, especially those living with chronic illnesses [12]. Pediatricians desire education about pediatric integrative medicine, yet few educational resources exist. The PIMR program was designed to fill this educational gap. Embedded into conventional training, it prepares pediatric residents to better serve the needs of their patients.

Preliminary results indicate that the PIMR curriculum targets identified knowledge gaps. The self-assessment and medical knowledge measures confirm the need for residents to receive exposure to this information. For example, few had awareness of IM approaches to common pediatric diagnoses such as asthma, attention deficit hyperactivity disorder, or migraine headaches. Self-assessment items specific to IM, such as knowledge of dietary supplements, received lower ratings, while more conventional topics, e.g., patient readiness to change, received higher ratings. Less than one-third had prior education or personal experience in IM. While deficits in skills and knowledge in IM would be expected upon starting residency, administration of the self-assessment and medical knowledge measures annually will allow us to track growing mastery of the curriculum content and identify content areas needing refinement.

Program implementation relies on the ability of residency programs to deliver IM education and to create a culture supportive of IM. Our initial site survey identified faculty background in IM and presence of affiliated IM practitioners as strengths across the sites. Further development is needed to support onsite IM educational activities. Site characteristics will be assessed annually to track evolution of the PIMR program's implementation and to identify characteristics associated with curriculum completion. Evaluation of the IMR program in family medicine to date indicates that the best predictors of successful program implementation are requiring program completion for graduation and including a greater number of onsite IM activities [11].

5. Conclusions

Success of the PIMR program will likely depend on residents' openness, interest, and readiness for IM training. In our survey, two-thirds of the residents expressed an interest in IM, and almost three-fourths were interested in applying IM after graduation. These findings, coupled with the self-assessment and medical knowledge results, suggest pediatric residents are interested, yet unschooled in IM when entering residency. The PIMR program provides a flexible, online curriculum that may satisfy resident interest and fill this knowledge gap. Evaluation of the curriculum is ongoing, and content will be refined in subsequent years to address identified learning gaps and feedback by participating residents and faculty.

Acknowledgments

The authors would like to thank the following for their contributions: Paula Cook, Research Specialist Senior, Grants and Contracts Manager, University of Arizona. Rhonda Hallquist, Instructional Web Developer, University of Arizona. Anna Esparham, University of Kansas Pediatrics Residency Program/University of Kansas Medical Center. Dana Gerstbacher, Stanford University School of Medicine/Children's Health Stanford. Brenda Golianu, Stanford University School of Medicine/Children's Health Stanford. Ann Ming Yeh, Stanford University School of Medicine/Children's Health Stanford. Callie Miller, Administrative Support, University of Arizona.

Funding was received from the David and Lura Lovell Foundation, The Weil Foundation, the Gerald J. and Rosalie E. Kahn Family Foundation, Inc. the John F. Long Foundation, the Resnick Foundation, and the Sampson Foundation.

Author Contributions

Hilary McClafferty, Sally Dodds, Audrey J. Brooks, and Patricia Lebensohn, conceived and designed the evaluations. Hilary McClafferty, Michelle G. Brenner, Melanie L. Brown, Paige Frazer, John D. Mark, Joy A. Weydert, and Graciela M.G. Wilcox performed the evaluations. Audrey Brooks, Sally Dodds, and Paula Cook analyzed the data. Hilary McClafferty, Sally Dodds, and Audrey Brooks wrote the paper. Patricia Lebensohn and Victoria Maizes provided editorial feedback.

Conflicts of Interest

The authors declare no conflict of interest.

References

1. Maizes, V.; Rakel, D.; Niemiec, C. Integrative Medicine and Patient-Centered Care. Institute of Medicine of the National Academies, 2009. Avaliable online: http://www.iom.edu/~/media/Files/Activity%20Files/Quality/IntegrativeMed/Integrative%20 Medicine%20and%20Patient%20Centered%20Care.pdf (accessed on 9 December 2014).
2. Kemper, K.J.; Vohra, S.; Walls, R.; The Task Force on Complementary and Alternative Medicine; Provisional Section on Complementary, Holistic, and Integrative Medicine. The use of complementary and alternative medicine in pediatrics. *Pediatrics.* **2008**, *122*, 1374–1386.
3. Vohra, S.; Surette, S.; Rosen, L.D.; Gardiner, P.; Kemper, K.J. Pediatric integrative medicine: Pediatrics' newest subspecialty? *BMC Pediatr.* **2012**, *15*, 123.

4. Institute of Medicine. Complementary and Alternative Medicine in the United States. Available online: http://www.iom.edu/reports/2005/complementary-and-alternative-medicine-in-the-united-states.aspx (accessed on 7 September 2014).

5. Maizes, V.; Schneider, C.; Bell, I.; Weil, A. Integrative medical education: Development and implementation of a comprehensive curriculum at the University of Arizona. *Acad. Med.* **2002**, *77*, 851–860.

6. Kligler, B.; Gordon, A.; Stuart, M.; Sierpina, V. Suggested curriculum guidelines on complementary and alternative medicine: recommendations of the Society of Teachers of Family Medicine Group on alternative medicine. *Fam. Med.* **2000**, *32*, 30–33.

7. Kligler, B.; Maizes, V.; Schachter, S.; Park, C.M.; Gaudet, T.; Benn, R.; Lee, R.; Remen, R.N.; Education Working Group; Consortium of Academic Health Centers for Integrative Medicine. Core competencies in integrative medicine for medical school curricula: A proposal. *Acad. Med.* **2004**, *79*, 521–531.

8. Ring, M.; Brodsky, M.; Low Dog, T.; Sierpina, V.; Bailey, M.; Locke, A.; Kogan, M.; Rindfleisch, J.A.; Saper, R. Developing and implementing core competencies for integrative medicine fellowships. *Acad. Med.* **2014**, *89*, 421–428.

9. American Board of Physician Specialties. Available online: http://www.abpsus.org/integrative-medicine (accessed on 9 December 2014).

10. Lebensohn, P.; Campos-Outcalt, D.; Senf, J.; Pugno, P.A. Experience with an optional 4-year residency: The University of Arizona Family Medicine Residency. *Fam. Med.* **2007**, *39*, 488–494.

11. Lebensohn, P.; Kligler, B.; Dodds, S.; Schneider, C.; Sroka, S.; Benn, R.; Cook, P.; Guerrera, M.; Dog, T.L.; Sierpina, V.; *et al.* Integrative medicine in residency education: Developing competency through online curriculum training. *J. Grad. Med. Educ.* **2012**, *4*, 76–82.

12. Birdee, G.S.; Phillips, R.S.; Davis, R.B.; Gardiner, P. Factors associated with pediatric use of complementary and alternative medicine. *Pediatrics* **2010**, *125*, 249–256.

13. Kemper, K.J.; O'Connor, K.G. Pediatricians' recommendations for complementary and alternative medical (CAM) therapies. *Ambul. Pediatr.* **2004**, *4*, 482–487.

14. Pediatric Milestone Project, page 99-104. Available online: http://acgme.org/acgmeweb/Portals/0/PDFs/Milestones/PediatricsMilestones.pdf (accessed on 9 December 2014).

15. Hicks, P.J.; Schumacher, D.J.; Benson, B.J.; Burke, A.E.; Englander, R.; Guralnick, S.; Ludwig, S.; Carraccio, C. The pediatrics milestones: Conceptual framework, guiding principles, and approach to development. *J. Grad. Med. Educ.* **2010**, *2*, 410–418.

MDPI AG
Klybeckstrasse 64
4057 Basel, Switzerland
Tel. +41 61 683 77 34
Fax +41 61 302 89 18
http://www.mdpi.com/

Children Editorial Office
E-mail: children@mdpi.com
http://www.mdpi.com/journal/children

www.ingramcontent.com/pod-product-compliance
Lightning Source LLC
Chambersburg PA
CBHW080133240326
41458CB00128B/6357